SpringerBriefs in Modern Perspectives on Disability Research

This book series on disability research is a comprehensive collection of research on disability and related issues. The series is designed to promote interdisciplinary collaboration and exchange, bringing together scholars and practitioners from different fields to share their perspectives and insights. Disability research is an interdisciplinary field that examines the social, cultural, historical, and political dimensions of disability. It encompasses a wide range of topics, including disability rights, accessibility, assistive technologies, healthcare, education, employment, and social welfare. Disability research scholars employ a range of theoretical and methodological approaches to understand the experiences of people with disabilities, as well as the ways in which disability intersects with other social identities such as race, gender, sexuality, and class.

The series seeks to advance knowledge and understanding of disability by publishing rigorous, innovative, and relevant research. It aims to promote disability rights and social justice by highlighting the ways in which people with disabilities are marginalized and discriminated against in society, and advocating for greater social inclusion and accessibility. The series also seeks to inform policy and practice by disseminating research findings that can help to shape policy decisions and contribute to positive social change.

Gabriel Bennett · Emma Goodall

The Role That Assistance Dogs Play in Supporting People with Disabilities

Springer

Gabriel Bennett
Independent Researcher
Klemzig, SA, Australia

Emma Goodall
Healthy Possibilities
Seaford, SA, Australia

ISSN 3004-9709 ISSN 3004-9717 (electronic)
SpringerBriefs in Modern Perspectives on Disability Research
ISBN 978-981-97-1491-9 ISBN 978-981-97-1492-6 (eBook)
https://doi.org/10.1007/978-981-97-1492-6

This Springer imprint is published by the registered company Springer Nature Singapore Pte Ltd.
The registered company address is: 152 Beach Road, #21-01/04 Gateway East, Singapore 189721, Singapore

Statement About the Usage of Artificial Intelligence

ChatGPT, a large language model artificial intelligence program developed by the company OpenAI, was used to enhance the clarity of the concepts articulated in this book. All other procedures that were used to create this research were performed by Dr. Gabriel Bennett and Dr. Emma Goodall.

Contents

About the Authors

Dr. Gabriel Bennett, Ph.D., the pen name for Dr. Matthew Bennett, holds a Ph.D. in Disability Studies from Flinders University, Australia. He has lectured in Disability Studies at Griffith University, Queensland. He has also advised the Australian Government's Autism CRC and has published articles for the *Journal of Autism and Developmental Disorders*. He is actively involved in supporting autistics and exploring key issues concerning disability.

Dr. Emma Goodall, Ph.D., is a senior industry researcher at Griffith University, an adjunct research fellow at the University of Southern Queensland, holds a Ph.D. in Education, focused on teaching students on the autism spectrum. She is an executive member of the Australian Society for Autism Research, independent researcher through Healthy Possibilities, a published author and keynote speaker in the areas of autism, sexuality and relationships, education, and interoception.

Together they have published several books, including:

1. Bennett, M., Webster, A. A., Goodall, E., & Rowland, S. (2019). *Life on the autism spectrum: Translating myths and misconceptions into positive futures.* Springer. https://doi.org/10.1007/978-981-13-3359-0
2. Bennett, M., Goodall, E., & Nugent, J. (2020). *Choosing Effective Support for People on the Autispm Spectrum: A Guide Based on Academic Perspectives and Lived Experience.* Routledge. https://doi.org/10.4324/9780367821975
3. Bennett, M., & Goodall, E. (2021). *Sexual Behaviours and Relationships of Autistics: A Scoping Review.* Springer International Publishing AG. https://doi.org/10.1007/978-3-030-65599-0
4. Bennett, M., & Goodall, E. (2021). *Employment of Persons with Autism: A Scoping Review.* Springer International Publishing AG. https://doi.org/10.1007/978-3-030-82174-6
5. Bennett, M., & Goodall, E. (2022). *Addressing Underserved Populations in Autism Spectrum Research: An Intersectional Approach.* Emerald Publishing Group. https://doi.org/10.1108/9781803824635

Acronyms

AAD	Autism-Assistance Dog
ADA	Americans with Disabilities Act
DSM	Diagnostic and Statistical Manual of Mental Disorders
ESD	Emotional Support Dog
ICF	International Classification of Functioning, Disability and Health
NDIS	National Disability Insurance Scheme
NSD	Neuro Service Dog
PAD	Psychiatric Assistance Dog
PCL	PTSD Checklist
PRISMA	Preferred Reporting Items for Systematic Reviews and Meta-Analyses
PTSD	Post-traumatic Stress Disorder
TBI	Traumatic Brain Injury
YOD	Young Onset Dementia

List of Figures

List of Tables

Chapter 1
Introduction

1.1 An Introduction to Dogs Assisting People with Disabilities

There are several strategies that can increase the prospect of people with disabilities participating in social, cultural, and economic opportunities and activities. For example, assistance technology has improved the quality of life for adults with intellectual disabilities in supported accommodation and the participation of people with disabilities in sport (Geppert et al., 2023; Morris et al., 2023). Changing societal attitudes and redesigning programs and physical structures, such as parks and shopping centres, are other strategies that can improve the quality of life of people with disabilities. For example, such strategies can help improve the participation of children with disabilities in physical activities (Wright et al., 2019). In conjunction with these strategies guide, assistance, support, and service dogs can also help some people with disabilities.

Sometimes the words '*guide*', '*assistance*', '*support*', and '*service*' are used interchangeably when describing dogs that can help people with disabilities. However, there are distinctions between these terms. To illustrate such distinctions Foltin and Glenk (2023) have offered the following definitions of assistance/service dogs and emotional support dogs (see Table 1.1). They have also explained the performance tasks and training that both types of dogs require (see Table 1.2).

G. Bennett and E. Goodall, *The Role That Assistance Dogs Play in Supporting People with Disabilities*, SpringerBriefs in Modern Perspectives on Disability Research,
https://doi.org/10.1007/978-981-97-1492-6_1

Table 1.1 Assistance dogs and Emotional Support Dogs (ESD): terminology, definitions, recipient

Definition/ recipient	Assistance dog/service dog	Emotional Support Dog (ESD)
Definition	*"An animal living with and highly trained to mitigate the impacts of the owner's disability, and with legal protections"*	An emotional support animal (ESA) may be an animal of any species (domestic, rare, or exotic) that provides some emotional or therapeutic support to an individual with a mental health condition or emotional disorder
	The Americans with Disabilities Act (ADA) defines service dogs as *"dogs that are individually trained to do work or perform tasks for people with disabilities"*	*"an animal who lives with and provides emotional benefit and/or support for the person, as confirmed by an appropriate qualified health care professional"*
	The U.S. Department of Justice uses the following definition: *"Service animals are defined as dogs that are individually trained to do work or perform tasks for people with disabilities. Service animals are working animals, not pets. The work or task a dog has been trained to provide must be directly related to the person's disability. Dogs whose sole function is to provide comfort or emotional support do not qualify as service animals under the ADA"*	
	"an animal who performs at least one identifiable task or behavior (not including any form of protection, comfort, or personal defense) to help a person with a disability to mitigate the impacts of that disability, and who is trained to a high standard of behavior and hygiene appropriate to access public spaces that are prohibited to most animals"	
Recipient	Individuals with a physical or psychological disability as defined by the Americans with Disabilities Act (ADA)	Any individual whose need is expressed in a request by a qualified physician, psychiatrist, or other mental health professional based upon a disability-related need

Source Foltin and Glenk (2023, p. 5)

Table 1.2 Assistance dogs and Emotional Support Dogs (ESD): performed tasks and training

Task	Assistance dog/service dog	Emotional Support Dog (ESD)
Performed tasks	Dogs perform at least one specific assistive task for individuals with a physical or psychological disability as defined by the Americans with Disabilities Act (ADA)	ESD provides companionship, affection, and support to people diagnosed with mental and emotional disabilities, autism, anxiety and panic attacks, depression, and various phobias. They provide comfort or emotional support by their mere presence
	Disability-mitigating tasks include the following: Opening and closing doors; turning light switches off and on; barking to indicate that help is needed; providing deep pressure; pulling a wheelchair; alerting to a medical crisis; providing assistance in a medical crisis; grounding their handler during a flashback; guiding their handler home during a dissociative episode; initiating tactile intervention when a handler experiences sensory overload; alleviating symptoms of hypervigilance	
Training	Service dogs are usually professionally trained but may also be trained by their owner. A service animal must be under the control of its handler. Under the ADA, service animals must be harnessed, leashed, or tethered, unless the individual's disability prevents using these devices or these devices interfere with the service animal's safe, effective performance of tasks. In that case, the individual must maintain control of the animal through voice, signal, or other effective controls	ESDs do not require specific training, licensing, registration, or certification and do not have to be trained for any particular task

Source Foltin and Glenk (2023, p. 7)

1.2 Relevance of This Book to the *Modern Perspectives on Disability Research* SpringerBrief Series

Disability research is an interdisciplinary field and scholars in this field examine the social, legal, cultural, historical, and political dimensions of disability. These scholars study a diverse range of topics, including disability rights, accessibility, inclusive design, the experiences of people with disabilities, assistive technology, healthcare, education, employment, and social welfare. They also study the ways in which disabilities, psychological, and medical conditions can intersect with other characteristics, such as race, gender, sexuality, and class. This SpringerBrief series,

Modern Perspectives on Disability Research, advances our knowledge about these topics.

A summary of the literature about the usage of assistance or support dogs among people with disabilities as well as people with psychological and/or medical conditions is presented in this book. It informs the reader about the benefits that such dogs can give specific groups and the challenges of using such dogs. By summarising and examining this literature this book fits the focus of this SpringerBrief series.

1.3 Research Questions

The primary objective of this book is to summarise the findings in the literature about the benefits and drawbacks that dogs can give people with disabilities and people with psychological and/or medical conditions. To achieve this objective four research questions were formulated before a search for studies on PubMed was conducted. Along with this study's eligibility criteria for citations, these research questions helped to determine what citations were or were not relevant to the study. These four research questions were:

1. Since 11 December 2018, what are the reported benefits and challenges in the literature associated with owning an assistance or service dog for people with specific disabilities?
2. What are the limitations in the reviewed literature about assistance or service dogs for people with disabilities?
3. Since 11 December 2018, what experiences have been documented in the literature about parents using an assistance or service dog for their child?
4. What are the views of professionals about the usage of assistance or service dogs that have been documented in the literature since 11 December 2018?

1.4 Search Procedures for Relevant Citations

On 11 December 2023, a search of PubMed was conducted to retrieve citations that could potentially answer the research questions. It was possible to search individual academic publishers (e.g., Routledge, Springer Nature, and SAGE). However, this approach was deemed to be ineffective because it would have involved a duplication of search procedures. Consequently, a search of PubMed was determined to be a more efficient approach for two reasons. First, the citations from different academic publishers are stored on PubMed. Thus, a single search of PubMed can retrieve citations from different publishers. Second, a search of PubMed enabled the identification of relevant studies from academic publishers that were unknown to the researchers.

A *Preferred Reporting Items for Systematic Reviews and Meta-Analyses* (PRISMA) approach was used to search and examine all citations retrieved from

PubMed. PRISMA is an established and widely used approach for collecting, examining, and identifying studies from a large sample of retrieved literature that answer a study's predetermined research questions. The PRISMA approach has five steps. These steps and their relation to this study are explained below.

- STEP ONE: The first step involved searching PubMed for studies about assistance, service, and guide dogs that supported people with disabilities, or medical, or psychological conditions. The search phrases (*'assistance dog*'* [Title]) OR (*'service dog*'* [Title]) OR (*'support dog*'* [Title]) OR (*'guide dog*'* [Title]) were used to retrieve studies.
- STEP TWO: The second step involved removing any duplicate records that were retrieved from the single search of PubMed. However, no duplicate records were identified.
- STEP THREE: The third step involved examining each retrieved citation's title and abstract to determine if it met the study's eligibility criteria. To be included in this study the citation had to have:
  - been published in English,
  - been published between 11 December 2018 to 11 December 2023, and
  - a sample of participants with disabilities and/or professionals who assist participants with disabilities and/or family members of people with disabilities.

    The citation could also be a literature review or a meta-analysis. However, citations that were retractions, corrections, letters to the editor, or commentaries were excluded.

    Of the 126 studies that were retrieved from the first step, 41 studies were deemed to be of interest.
- STEP FOUR: The fourth step involved reading the entire text of the 41 studies that were provisionally deemed to answer one or more of the research questions. All 41 studies were deemed to answer one or more of the research questions.
- STEP FIVE: The fifth and final step involved identifying, examining, summarising, and explaining the results from the 41 studies that were retained from the fourth step in the PRISMA analysis process (see Fig. 1.1).

1.5 Methodological Strengths and Weaknesses of This Study

1.5.1 Methodological Strengths

1.5.1.1 Publication of the Study's Dataset

The *'reproducibility crisis'* refers to the inability to validate a study's findings because the dataset is not published along with the study and/or the methodological procedures used to conduct the study, including examining the dataset, are not clearly described

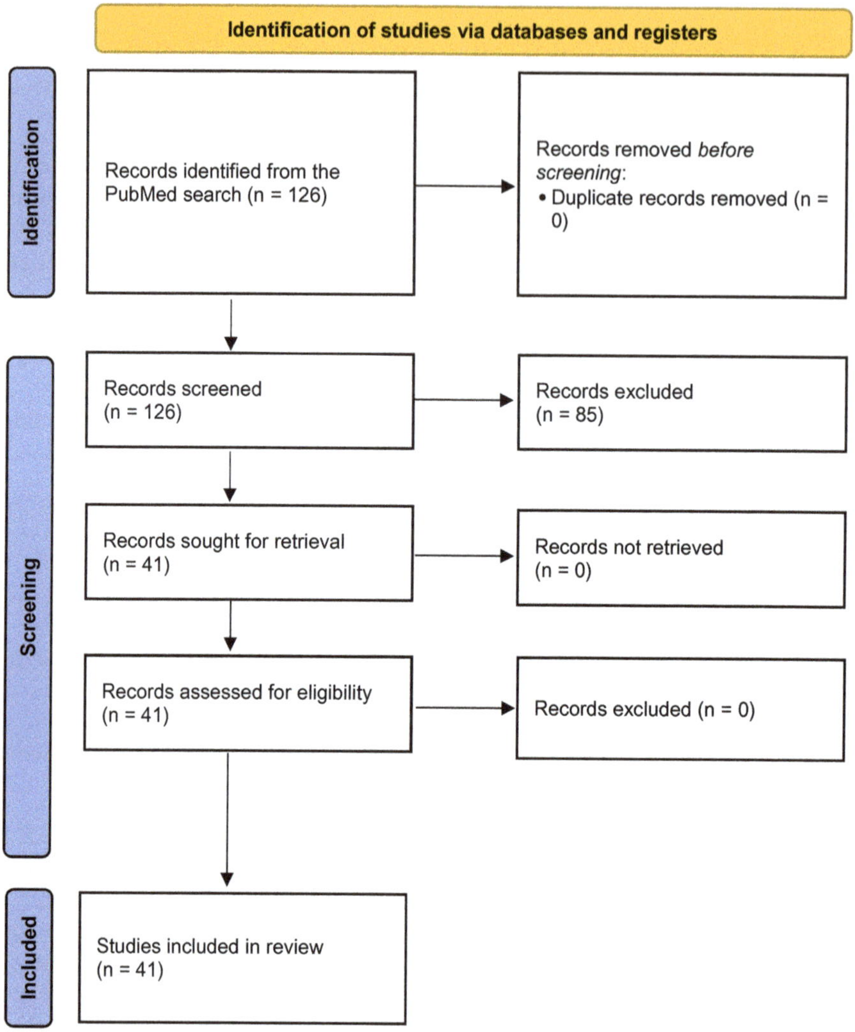

Fig. 1.1 Preferred reporting items for systematic reviews and meta-analyses (PRISMA) flow diagram. *Source* Page, M. J., McKenzie, J. E., Bossuyt, P. M., Boutron, I., Hoffmann, T. C., Mulrow, C. D., Shamseer, L., Tetzlaff, J. M., Akl, E. A., Brennan, S. E., Chou, R., Glanville, J., Grimshaw, J. M., Hróbjartsson, A., Lalu, M. M., Li, T., Loder, E. W., Mayo-Wilson, E., McDonald, S., McGuinness, L. A., … Moher, D. (2021). The PRISMA 2020 statement: An updated guideline for reporting systematic reviews. BMJ (Clinical research ed.), 372, n71. https://doi.org/10.1136/bmj.n71

(Bennett, 2023). To mitigate the prospect of this study succumbing to this crisis the dataset of all the records generated from the PubMed search is published (see Appendix A). This dataset gives future researchers the opportunity to repeat the same analysis to either confirm or disprove the conclusions reported.

1.5.1.2 Wide Range of Search Terms

A relatively large number of keywords were used to search PubMed so that the maximum number of studies about the utility of dogs for people with disabilities, psychological, or medical conditions could be retrieved. Despite this search approach, it is possible that some articles were not retrieved from the PubMed search using these keywords.

1.5.2 Methodological Weaknesses

1.5.2.1 Only Accessing Studies from PubMed

All articles that were examined for this study were obtained from a single search of PubMed, that occurred on 11 December 2023. PubMed was used because it contained many relevant studies about disability. It was also used because it indexed studies that were published by several reputable academic publishers (e.g., SAGE, Routledge, Springer Nature) and several reputable journals about disability (e.g., Disability and Rehabilitation, Qualitative Health Research). Despite this approach, it is possible that there were studies that were not included in the analysis because they were not published on PubMed. However, the large number of relevant articles retrieved from the PubMed search mitigated this methodological limitation.

1.5.2.2 Restricting the Search Terms to the Article's Title

To guarantee that the most relevant studies were discovered, the article's title had to contain one of the following search terms *'assistance dog'*, *'service dog'*, *'support dog'*, and *'guide dog'*. Despite this approach, it is possible that some articles that would have been relevant for this study were not retrieved from PubMed because the search term was instead embedded within the article's abstract and/or full text instead of its title. However, the prospect of this occurrence was deemed to be rare. Nevertheless, it cannot be ruled out that some articles may not have been identified.

1.5.2.3 Only English Studies Were Examined

Only articles published in English were examined for this study. Consequently, articles that were published in other languages that contained relevant information were not examined. Due to this situation, their contributions to this study were not included.

1.6 Intended Audience for This Book

This book has been written for many different audiences, including:

- *Researchers and Academics:* Researchers, scholars, and academics in the fields of psychology, disability studies, human–animal interaction, and related disciplines would be interested in exploring the existing research and evidence summarised in this book.
- *Healthcare Professionals:* Healthcare professionals, such as doctors, therapists, and rehabilitation specialists, who work with people with disabilities would be interested in understanding the potential benefits and applications of dogs as a complementary intervention in supporting their patients.
- *Assistance Dog Organisations and Trainers:* Organisations and professionals involved in training and working with dogs that assist people with disabilities would find this book valuable. They would be interested in gaining insights into the current research and best practices in the field to enhance their training programs and support services.
- *Individuals with Disabilities and Their Families:* People with disabilities and their families who are considering or currently using dogs as part of their support system would find this book informative and relevant. It can provide them with a comprehensive understanding of the potential benefits, considerations, and experiences associated with dogs.
- *Policy Makers and Advocacy Groups:* Government officials, policymakers, and advocacy groups focused on disability rights and services would be interested in understanding the evidence-based benefits and implications of assistance dogs. This book can inform policy discussions and decisions regarding the integration of dogs into healthcare, accessibility, and support systems.

1.7 Benefits of This Book

This book will provide many benefits for the reader, including:

- *Comprehensive Scoping Review:* This book presents a comprehensive scoping review that summarises the existing research about the role of dogs in supporting people with disabilities. It provides a comprehensive overview of the current state of knowledge in this field.
- *Evidence-Based Approach:* The content of this book is grounded in evidence-based research, ensuring that readers receive reliable and credible information. It critically examines research studies and their methodologies, providing a balanced and informed perspective.
- *Inclusive Coverage of Assistance Dog Types:* This book covers various types of assistance dogs, including guide dogs, hearing dogs, service dogs for physical disabilities, and psychiatric service dogs. It explores the specific roles and benefits

of each type, offering a comprehensive understanding of the diverse ways dogs can support people with disabilities.

- *Focus on Outcomes and Benefits:* This book emphasises the outcomes and benefits that dogs can give people with disabilities, such as increased independence, improved wellbeing, and enhanced social interaction. Readers will gain insights into the real-life impact of such dogs on the lives of people with disabilities.
- *Future Directions and Implications:* This book explores future directions, challenges, and considerations related to dogs that help people with disabilities. It discusses the implications for research, practice, and policy. Readers will gain valuable insights into the evolving landscape of this topic.

1.8 Description of Upcoming Chapters

1.8.1 Chapter 2—Results in the Existing Literature

In Chap. 2, the results in the selected citations from the PubMed search are presented. The focus of this chapter is on explaining the impact of owning an assistance or service dog for people with disabilities and their families. These results are categorised into three themes, which are: (1) Consequences associated with owning an assistance or service dog, (2) Documented experiences about parents using an assistance or service dog for their children, and (3) Views of professionals about the usage of assistance or service dogs.

1.8.2 Chapter 3—Limitations of Current Studies

In Chap. 3, the limitations in the studies presented in Chap. 2 are outlined. These limitations include that the study's sample size was small and that participants had become accustomed to the survey instruments. The purpose of this chapter is to inform the reader about the current limitations in our research about the benefits and drawbacks that people with disabilities obtain from dogs, whether they be assistance dogs, service dogs, or emotional support dogs.

1.8.3 Chapter 4—Directions for Research in the Future

In Chap. 4, the limitations in the current research that were presented in Chap. 3 are collated and summarised. The purpose of this exercise is to highlight the limitations that are commonly shared between studies and to outline potential solutions to these identified limitations. Additionally, in this chapter, a reiteration of this study's design (e.g., study's aims and the study's methodological limitations) is presented.

References

Bennett, M. (2023). *Applying metascientific principles to autism Research.* Springer Nature.

Foltin, S., & Glenk, L. M. (2023). Current perspectives on the challenges of implementing assistance dogs in human mental health care. *Veterinary Sciences, 10*(1), 62. https://doi.org/10.3390/vetsci10010062

Geppert, A., Smith, E. M., Haslett, D., Wong, J., Ebuenyi, I. D., & MacLachlan, M. (2023). Assistive technology to promote participation in sport for people with disabilities. *Studies in Health Technology and Informatics, 306*, 191–198. https://doi.org/10.3233/SHTI230618

Morris, B., Warren, A., Bradwell, H., & Noonan, M. (2023). Barriers and facilitators of the adoption and use of assistive technology for adults with an intellectual disability who live in supported accommodation: A mixed methods systematic review protocol. *JBI Evidence Synthesis, 21*(6), 1259–1269. https://doi.org/10.11124/JBIES-22-00313

Wright, A., Roberts, R., Bowman, G., & Crettenden, A. (2019). Barriers and facilitators to physical activity participation for children with physical disability: Comparing and contrasting the views of children, young people, and their clinicians. *Disability and Rehabilitation, 41*(13), 1499–1507. https://doi.org/10.1080/09638288.2018.1432702

Chapter 2
Results in the Existing Literature

2.1 Consequences of Owning an Assistance or Service Dog

2.1.1 Veterans and Ex-military Service People

An examination of the citations that were collected after searching PubMed yielded 15 studies about the utility of assistance or service dogs for military veterans (Hansen et al., 2023; Jensen et al., 2021, 2022; LaFollette et al., 2019; Leighton et al., 2022; McLaughlin & Hamilton, 2019; Nieforth et al., 2022c; Richerson et al., 2023; Rodriguez et al., 2020c, 2021; Sherman et al., 2023; Shiroff et al., 2022; van Houtert et al., 2022; Whitworth et al., 2019; Woodward et al., 2021). What follows now is a description of each study's design and its results.

Hansen et al. (2023) measured over a one-year duration the effectiveness of two Australian PTSD assistance dog programs in alleviating PTSD and mental health symptoms among veterans. To achieve this objective they measured the PTSD and mental health symptoms of 44 veterans that had been matched with an assistance dog. Based on the data collected, compared to the baseline measurements, reductions in all mental health problems were statistically significant at the 3-month follow-up. These reductions were also sustained at both the 6-month and 12-month follow-up time points. Among those who completed the waitlist-baseline evaluation ($n = 23$), minor reductions in stress and depression were observed prior to receiving their dog while they were waiting. However, comparing the waitlist-baseline measurements to the 3-month follow-up measurements showed greater reductions across all mental health indicators.

Psychiatric service dogs are increasingly being used as an additional intervention for those with PTSD. While preliminary evidence suggests that veterans who interact with a psychiatric service dog may experience a reduction in their PTSD symptom severity, the mechanisms behind this relationship are not yet clear. To address this

G. Bennett and E. Goodall, *The Role That Assistance Dogs Play in Supporting People with Disabilities*, SpringerBriefs in Modern Perspectives on Disability Research,
https://doi.org/10.1007/978-981-97-1492-6_2

gap, Jensen et al. (2022) conducted a longitudinal study with 82 post-9/11 military members or veterans and their PTSD service dogs. Their study aimed to:

- Evaluate service dog characteristics as potential predictors of therapy efficacy,
- Assess dog and human characteristics as potential predictors of veteran–dog bond, and
- Explore potential mechanisms for mental health outcomes.

The findings from their study indicated that most psychiatric service dog attributes did not have a significant impact on the mental health outcomes of veterans. However, a psychiatric service dog with less levels of excitability was linked to lower severity of PTSD symptoms at the follow-up time point. Their study also revealed that stronger bonds between a veteran and their psychiatric service dog were linked to a calmer and composed temperament exhibited by the dog. Their study also demonstrated that veterans with poor mental health outcomes were more likely to rely on their psychiatric service dog for initiating social interactions and making new acquaintances.

Cross-sectional studies have demonstrated that service dogs can have a significant impact on reducing the severity of PTSD symptoms among veterans. However, to measure PTSD symptoms these studies relied on the PTSD checklist (PCL) from the fourth edition of the *Diagnostic and Statistical Manual of Mental Disorders* (DSM). Using a version of the PCL based on the fifth edition of the DSM (PCL-5), Jensen et al. (2021) aimed to replicate and advance the findings from these previous cross-sectional studies. They sampled 186 military members and veterans, of which 112 had received a service dog to help them manage their PTSD, while the other 74 were on a waitlist to receive a service dog. After demographic variables were mitigated, they discovered that having a service dog helped lower PTSD symptom severity, both in total scores and within each PCL-5 symptom cluster. This study's results support prior research and give credence to the notion that service dogs can be an extra support for military members and veterans with PTSD. These outcomes underscore the need for more clinical research about using service dogs to help military members and veterans manage their PTSD.

Military veterans are increasingly interacting with psychiatric service dogs to help them manage their PTSD. LaFollette et al. (2019) explored the associations between PTSD severity service dog behaviour, training methods for service dogs, and the veteran-service dog bond in a population of military veterans with PTSD. They sampled 111 post-9/11 military veterans with PTSD who interacted with a psychiatric service dog that was provided by a national service dog provider. The veterans completed an online survey about their training methods, severity of PTSD symptoms, behaviours of service dogs, and the bond between human–animal. Most service dogs came from dog shelters or rescues and were mainly Labrador Retriever purebreds or mixes of various breeds. They divided the training methods into five categories, which were:

- Positive reinforcement (e.g., physical praise),
- Negative punishment (e.g., ignoring the dog),
- Positive punishments (e.g., verbal correction),
- Dominance (e.g., alpha roll), and
- Broad-based (e.g., co-sleeping).

The use of positive reinforcement and bond-based methods were associated with more positive outcomes, such as higher closeness to their service dog, increased attachment behaviour, and playfulness. However, the use of positive punishment was associated with more negative outcomes, such as less closeness with their service dog, more fear, less eye contact, and less trainability. Their study concluded that educating service dog organisations and recipients about the impacts of training methods could be beneficial for service dog efficacy and welfare (LaFollette et al., 2019).

Leighton et al. (2022) published a literature review about the use of psychiatric assistance dogs for military veterans with PTSD. They attempted to summarise the main characteristics of the literature, evaluate its quality, and collate the main results. A total of 41 articles met their inclusion criteria, of which 29 were peer-reviewed articles and 12 were unpublished dissertations (see Tables 2.1 and 2.2). Most articles were quantitative (53%), while 41% were qualitative, and 6% used mixed methods. The quantitative articles examined reported significant improvements in PTSD severity, mental health, and social health. However, it was inconclusive if psychiatric assistance dogs helped improve physical health or quality of life. Their review supports the view that psychiatric assistance dogs can help mitigate PTSD severity among veterans.

Few studies have explored if service dogs can help military veterans with PTSD increase their participation in daily activities. McLaughlin and Hamilton (2019) explored the experiences of a sample of Australian military veterans with PTSD who had been paired with a service dog. Seven participants were recruited from a veteran's support organisation and two semi-structured focus group sessions were conducted. They identified several themes related to the experience of Australian military veterans with PTSD interacting with a service dog, including isolation, safety, lifeline, reconnection, and challenges. These participants explained that having a service dog improved their sense of safety and their ability to manage their PTSD. This resulted in a variety of positive changes, such as better sleep quality, improved emotional regulation, reduced anxiety, better anger management, and a decrease in alcohol and prescription medication misuse, and reduced suicide ideation. As a result, participants were able to improve their relationships and engage in more meaningful daily activities. This study highlights the potential benefits of service dogs for veterans with military service-related PTSD (McLaughlin & Hamilton, 2019).

Nieforth et al. (2022c) compared the experiences of veterans using a service dog for PTSD to the expectations of veterans who were on a waitlist for a service dog for their PTSD. A total of 128 United States post-9/11 veterans with PTSD were recruited from *K9s for Warriors*, a non-profit service dog provider, of which 69 used a service dog for PTSD and 59 were in the waitlist group. They reported that:

Table 2.1 Non-veteran participant studies: participants, design, and outcomes

Study	Participants (n)	Design	Outcomes
Peer-reviewed			
Woodward et al. (2021)	Veterans training SDs, inpatient program (54)	Repeated measures (ABAB)	✓ Canine's presence associated with ↓ negative, ↑ positive affect; stronger effect with greater PTSD severity – Negative affect ↓ with time in program; effect of canine's presence on negative affect also ↓ with time
van Houtert et al. (2021)	SDs (19)	Cross-sectional	✓ Psychiatric service dogs for veterans with PTSD do not appear stressed when training and performing tasks – Cortisol ↑ after arrival at training centre and after 45 m of play
Whitworth et al. (2020)	Partners of veterans in SD training program (15)	Qualitative	✓ Benefits of supportive relationships (human and dog); better partner relationships via ↑ symptom management; partners help maintain participation in program – Propose attachment theory-based model: new and improved relationships via SD program forms "relational bridge" leading to ↑ resilience ✘ Ongoing relational challenges; limited support for own needs; challenges with public understanding; partners have own trauma; caregiver burden
McCall et al. (2020)	Partners of veterans with SDs (37) and on WL (23)	Cross-sectional + Qualitative	✓ More benefits than challenges; ↑ resilience and companionship; ↓ anger, social isolation, and work impairment – No significant differences in functioning between groups ✘ Unwanted attention in public; financial cost; adjusting to changed roles
Vincent et al. (2017a)	SD trainers (12) Veterans with SD (1) Veteran advocates (4) Medical professionals (3) Standards board (1)	Qualitative	• Developed theory-oriented logic model: "Sequence of needs and experience that lead PTSD patients to seek a [Psychiatric Service Dog]"

(continued)

Table 2.1 (continued)

Study	Participants (n)	Design	Outcomes
Dissertations			
Genbauffe (2020)	Psychotherapists (3)	Qualitative	– All participants have positive attitudes towards pet dogs ✘ Consider use of SD as potential safety behaviour; SD may interfere with natural recovery process; concerned with SD fraud/lack of certification
Tilvaldiev (2019)	SD trainers (11) Mental health professionals (6)	Qualitative	• Developed proposed standards for placement of SDs and veterans with PTSD (23 items)

Note Ordered in reverse chronological order within each category (peer-reviewed, dissertation). SD service dog. WL waitlist to receive service dog. PCL-5 PTSD Checklist for DSM-5. ✓ Positive outcome; – Neutral or null outcome; ✘ Negative outcome; • Theory-based framework or protocol result. ↑ increased; ↓ decreased
Source Leighton et al. (2022, p. 8)

> The most commonly reported benefits from Veterans with service dogs were the service dog's ability to help Veterans get out into the community as well as the positivity that the service dog brought into Veterans' lives. The most commonly mentioned drawback from Veterans with service dogs was the increased attention they received in public due to the presence of the service dog. (Nieforth et al., 2022c, p. 12)

Currently, there is a need for a clear understanding of the components of the PTSD service dog intervention for military veterans with PTSD. Rodriguez et al. (2022) recruited 217 post-9/11 military veterans with PTSD, of which 134 had a service dog and 83 were in the waitlist group. The results showed that from the perspective of the participants the most important and often used trained tasks were the dog's calming behaviours and interrupting anxiety. However, they reported that veterans who felt emotionally attached to their service dogs tended to utilise their dogs' trained task more frequently. On the other hand, veterans who had owned their service dogs for an extended period used trained tasks less frequently. Additionally, veterans who were on the waiting list for a service dog reported greater expectations about the use and importance of trained tasks than those who already had a service dog.

The therapeutic benefits that service dogs have on the medication usage of veterans with PTSD have largely been unexplored. To address this gap, Rodriguez et al. (2021) investigated the impact of PTSD service dogs on medication usage among post-9/11 military veterans with PTSD. They recruited 96 post-9/11 military veterans with PTSD from a single service dog provider, of which 52 had a service dog for PTSD and 44 were on a waitlist. Medication regimens and changes were reported by participants via an online survey. The results showed that having a service dog did not have any significant effects on overall self-reported medication use or any specific medication category. However, veterans with a service dog were more likely to report that their

Table 2.2 Study characteristics

Study	Design	Control	N	PTSD measure	Outcomes
Peer-reviewed					
Jensen et al. (2021)	Cross-sectional	WL	186 SD: 112 WL: 74	PCL-5 ✓	✓ ↓ PCL scores – PCL scores above diagnostic cutoff. No association with time since placement
Nieforth et al. (2023)	Qualitative	–	101 SD: 67 P: 34	CAPS-5	✓ ↓ PTSD symptoms; ↑ emotional reserves. Aid communication and emotional regulation within family. Trained tasks ↑ independence – Recommendations to providers/mental health teams ✘ ↑ relational load for partner
Nieforth et al. (2022c)	Qualitative	WL	128 SD: 69 WL: 59	PCL-C	✓ ↑ community engagement, QoL; ↓ anxiety. Trained tasks beneficial, and benefit extends beyond tasks via bond – Gap between expectations and reality ✘ ↑ challenges in public[a] and when travelling
Rodriguez et al. (2021)	Cross-sectional	WL	96 SD: 52 WL: 44	PCL-C	✓ ↓ PCL scores. More likely to report decrease in medications – No effect when comparing self-reported medication list

(continued)

Table 2.2 (continued)

Study	Design	Control	N	PTSD measure	Outcomes
Williamson et al. (2021)	Single subject (AB) + Qualitative	Pre-Post (12 m)	5	PCL-5 ✓	✓ Clinically (not statistically) significant ↓ PCL scores. Trained tasks ↑ independence, ↓ PTSD symptoms. Report ↓ opioid use – No effect on DUSI-R SU score ✘ ↑ challenges in public[a]. Frustrations with training/bonding process
Galsgaard and Eskelund (2020)	Single subject (AB)	Pre-Post (16 m)	4	PCL-C	✓ ↑ social engagement, sense of agency. ↓ trauma-related intrusion PTSD symptoms – Impact on overall PTSD symptoms unclear – ↓ PCL scores for 2 of 4 participants
Husband et al. (2020)	Qualitative	–	4	–	✓ ↓ substance use, PTSD symptoms. ↓ or no change in prescription medication – No change in opiate use
Lessard et al. (2020)	Pre-post	Pre-Post (9 m)	18	PCL-M ✓	✓ ↑ moderate physical activity, steps per day (actigraphy). ↑ sleep (self-report). ↓ median PCL score, depression – No change in sedentary behaviours, sleep (actigraphy)

(continued)

Table 2.2 (continued)

Study	Design	Control	N	PTSD measure	Outcomes
Richerson et al. (2020)	Randomised control	ESA	227 SD: 114 ES: 113	CAPS-5 PCL-5 ✓	✓ ↓ disability, ↑ QoL for *both* groups. ↓ PCL score, ↓ suicidal behaviours and ideation for SD group. Based on CAPS-5, PTSD absent in 28% of SD group at 15 months (0% absent at baseline) – Unable to reject null hypothesis for primary and most secondary outcomes ✘ PTSD symptoms worsened from baseline up until pairing
Rodriguez et al. (2020c)	Cross-sectional	WL	217 SD: 134 WL: 83	PCL-5 ✓	✓ ↓ PCL scores. All trained tasks beneficial. Untrained tasks more important on average – ↓ task usage with time; ↑ task usage with stronger bond. Trained tasks least helpful for amnesia, risk-taking. Gap between expectations and reality ✘ Tasks least helpful for difficulty remembering trauma, engaging in reckless behaviour

(continued)

Table 2.2 (continued)

Study	Design	Control	N	PTSD measure	Outcomes
Lafollette et al. (2019)	Cross-sectional	–	111	PCL-5 ✓	✓ Bond is mutually strong. More frequent + R/bond-based training associated with stronger bond – No association between PTSD severity and bond or SD behaviour or character ✘ More frequent + P training associated with weaker bond
McLaughlin and Hamilton (2019)	Qualitative	–	7	–	✓ ↓ isolation, anxiety, substance use, suicidal ideation. ↑ feeling of safety, sleep quality, emotional regulation ✘ Financial (veterinary care). Anticipation of grief due to dog lifespan
Scotland-Coogan (2019a)	Qualitative	–	15	–	✓ ↓ anger. ↑ social engagement. Improved relationships
Scotland-Coogan (2019b)	Qualitative	–	15	–	✓ ↓ symptom severity, anxiety, insomnia, nightmares
Whitworth et al. (2019)	Non-randomised control	WL	30 SD: 15 WL: 15	Tsi-2	✓ ↓ PTSD symptoms, depression, anger. Improved relationships. ↑ social engagement – No change in somatisation, understanding/communication, self-care, life activities
Crowe et al. (2018a)	Qualitative	–	9	–	✓ Constant, calming presence. ↑ social and community engagement

(continued)

Table 2.2 (continued)

Study	Design	Control	N	PTSD measure	Outcomes
Crowe et al. (2018b)	Qualitative	–	6	–	✓ ↑ safety (physical), peace of mind, healthy behaviours. Bond exceeds expectations. Improved relationships overall ✘ Lack of acceptance, strained or lost relationships in some cases
Lessard et al. (2018)	Qualitative	–	10	–	✓ Trained tasks beneficial. Companionship. ↓ medication, PTSD symptoms. ↑ social, community engagement – Recommendations for providers ✘ Stress (veterinary care). ↑ challenges in public[a]. Issues in acquisition process
O'Haire and Rodriguez (2018)	Non-randomised control	WL	141 SD: 75 WL: 66	PCL-C	✓ ↓ PCL score, depression, absenteeism due to health. ↑ QoL, social functioning – No effect on physical health, employment status. No effect on treatment participation
Rodriguez et al. (2018)	Cross-sectional	WL	73 SD: 45 WL: 28	PCL-C ✓	✓ More typical cortisol awakening response. ↓ anxiety, anger, sleep disturbances, substance use – No effect on sleep quality. No association between PTSD severity and cortisol awakening response

(continued)

Table 2.2 (continued)

Study	Design	Control	N	PTSD measure	Outcomes
Yarborough et al. (2018)	Qualitative	–	55 SD: 41 P: 8 T: 6	Clinician report	✓ Trained tasks ↓ PTSD symptoms. ↑ social, community engagement. ↓ suicidality, medication use – Emphasise importance of preparation. Partners may have mixed feelings ✘ Training is stressful and tiring. Benefits take time. ↑ challenges in public[a]
Kloep et al. (2017)	Pre-post	Pre-Post (6 m)	13	PCL-S ✓	✓ ↓ PCL score, depression, anger. ↑ sleep quality, perceived social support, QoL
Vincent et al. (2017b)	Pre-post	Pre-Post (3 m)	15	PCL-M ✓	✓ ↓ PCL score, depression. ↑ sleep quality – No effect on QoL and social engagement
Yarborough et al. (2017)	Cross-sectional	WL	78 SD: 24 WL: 54	PCL-C ✓	✓ Tasks beneficial. ↓ PCL score, depression. ↑ happiness, QoL. Improved mental health overall – No effect on physical health, activity level
Dissertations					
Floore-Guetschow (2020)	Qualitative	–	7	–	✓ ↑ enjoyment of day-to-day life, social and community engagement. ↓ PTSD symptoms – Some re-engaged/ continued mental health treatments; others discontinued ✘ Anticipation of grief due to dog lifespan. ↑ challenges in public[a]

(continued)

Table 2.2 (continued)

Study	Design	Control	N	PTSD measure	Outcomes
Hansen (2019)	Cross-sectional	Combat versus noncombat	64	PCL-5	✓ Task usage positively associated with PTSD severity – Insecure attachment style positively associated with task usage
Parenti (2019)	Repeated measures (ABCDE)	Dog (SD/pet) present/absent	6	PCL-5	✓ ↓ heart rate, negative affect in presence of dog. Negative affect significantly lower for SD condition – Stress indicators declined overall throughout session. No effect on heart rate, mental workload
Kegel (2016)	Cross-sectional	V	66 SD: 43 V: 23	PCL-M	✓ ↑ QoL (social engagement, creative expression) – No association with PCL score, substance use, other QoL areas ✘ ↑ difficulty falling and staying asleep
Kopicki (2016)	Cross-sectional	WL	18 SD:12 WL: 6	PCL-M	✓ ↓ PCL (hyperarousal subscale) – No effect on other PCL areas. Placement length not associated with PTSD symptoms, sleep quality
Brown (2015)	Qualitative	–	1	–	✓ ↑ sense of physical and emotional safety. ↓ medication, PTSD symptoms Tasks beneficial ✘ ↑ challenges in public[a]

(continued)

Table 2.2 (continued)

Study	Design	Control	N	PTSD measure	Outcomes
Hyde (2015)	Cross-sectional + Qualitative	–	7	PCL-5	✓ ↑ hope, social and community engagement, routine – No effect on PCL scores ✘ ↑ challenges in public[a]. Burden of care. Little planning around retirement
Marston (2015)	Cross-sectional	WL	18 SD:12 WL: 6	-	– No effect on QoL. No association with time since pairing
Moore (2014)	Qualitative	–	8	–	✓ ↓ PTSD symptoms. ↑ sense of safety, social engagement. Trained tasks, bond both beneficial – Some participants integrated SD in therapy ✘ ↑ challenges in public[a]
Newton (2014)	Qualitative	–	6	–	✓ ↓ PTSD symptoms. ↑ community and social engagement – Emphasise importance of working with a good organisation ✘ ↑ challenges in public[a]. Frustrations with training experiences

Note Ordered by most recent to least recent within each group. SD Veterans with service dogs. WL Waitlist to receive service dog. ES Emotional support dog. Pre Preplacement. V Veterans not on waitlist nor partnered with service dog. P Partner. T Service dog trainer. PCL PTSD Checklist (-C Civilian; -M Military; -S Specific; -5 for DSM-5). CAPS Clinician-Administered PTSD Scale. TSI-2 Trauma Symptom Inventory-2. PCL ✓ Clinically significant improvement in mean score; PCL Mean score change not clinically significant; Italics indicates time points. No symbol: Mean score change not reported. ✓ Positive outcome; – Neutral or null outcome; ✘ Negative outcome. ↑ increased; ↓ decreased. QoL Quality of Life. DUSI-R SU Drug Use Screening Inventory Revised Substance Use Subscale. + R Positive reinforcement. + P Positive punishment

[a]Challenges in public may include access issues, stigma, and unwanted attention

Source Leighton et al. (2022, pp. 9–11)

doctor had decreased or stopped prescribing medications since interacting with their service dog than those on the waitlist.

Sherman et al. (2023) conducted a mixed-method longitudinal study to examine the effectiveness of *Operation K9* assistance dogs among 16 veterans with PTSD, focusing on their impact on suicidality, PTSD, depression, and anxiety from baseline to 12 months post-matching. Self-reported measures were collected from participants before receiving their assistance dog (i.e., baseline) and at three time points (i.e., 3, 6, and 12 months) after matching had occurred. The severity of every PTSD case was measured using the *Clinician-Administered PTSD Scale for DSM-5*. At three months post-matching veterans also participated in a semi-structured interview. While the proportion of veterans reporting suicidality decreased, the occurrence of veterans disclosing that they had suicidal thoughts between time points was not significant. However, there was a significant effect over time on PTSD, depression, and anxiety symptoms. An analysis of the qualitative data revealed three major themes, which were (1) assistance dogs as life changes, (2) assistance dogs as constant companions, and (3) facilitators of social engagement. The results suggest that assistance dogs can positively impact important areas of daily life and support veterans in accessing services, transportation, education, employment, and developing diverse social and community connections, which are essential prerequisites for good health.

As a relatively new area of research with limited empirical evidence, it is unclear if a service dog genuinely alleviates the symptoms of PTSD. To investigate the potential impact of service dogs on veterans and first responders with PTSD, van Houtert et al. (2022) examined both the subjective and psychological parameters among 65 people who were divided into four groups. They were veterans and first responders with PTSD and:

1. A service dog ($n = 20$),
2. A companion dog ($n = 10$), or
3. Without a dog ($n = 12$).

The final group was a control group without PTSD ($n = 23$). Their results showed that, in comparison to those who interacted with a companion dog, veterans and first responders with PTSD who interacted with a service dog reported significantly fewer PTSD-related symptoms, better sleep quality, and greater overall wellbeing. Participants with a service dog also reported experiencing fewer PTSD-related symptoms than those without a service dog. While more research on the use of psychological measures is needed, their study suggests that owning a service dog can have a positive impact on subjective wellbeing, sleep quality, and symptoms relating to PTSD.

Whitworth et al. (2019) investigated the effectiveness of a 14-week service dog training program in central Florida for military veterans with PTSD. Thirty veterans with PTSD were evenly divided into one of two groups: an intervention group ($n = 15$) and a waitlist group ($n = 15$). All participants completed the 136-item *Trauma Symptom Inventory-2.0* and the 36-item *World Health Organisation Disability Assessment Schedule-2* before and after the study. The results showed that the intervention group demonstrated significant reductions in PTSD symptoms and reduced intra- and inter-personal difficulties related to psychological trauma compared to the control group. Their study adds to the growing evidence that for some veterans with PTSD the use of service dogs may be a viable complementary or alternative treatment option. Consequently, practitioners may want to consider referring their veteran clients with PTSD to accredited service dog programs to supplement traditional therapy approaches.

Although service dogs are a popular treatment option for treating PTSD, there has been limited empirical evaluation about their efficacy. Woodward et al. (2021) evaluated the utility of a service dog program at the United States Department of Veterans Affairs residential PTSD treatment program. They compared the phenotypic markers of participants when they were accompanied by their service dog versus when they were not. Their study involved 54 veterans over a period of two to six weeks. The results they collected support prior reports that service dogs can reduce PTSD symptoms. However, their results should be carefully endorsed considering that their study was brief and conducted in an artificial environment.

Shiroff et al. (2022) performed qualitative research intended to contribute to the existing knowledge supporting the advantages of service dogs as an additional treatment approach for veterans dealing with PTSD and/or traumatic brain injury (TBI). For their study, open-ended, semi-structured interviews were conducted with a sample of veterans ($n = 10$) who were utilising service dogs as a form of treatment for either PTSD and/or TBI. Their analysis of the transcripts revealed four primary themes and several sub-themes. These primary themes included functional status, the influence of a service dog, the service dog's ability to recognise symptoms of PTSD and/or TBI, and the obstacles associated with obtaining a service dog. Some participants expressed the view that bonding with the service dog notably enhanced their social interactions and served as a beneficial component to treatment approaches for managing their PTSD and/or TBI. Based on these results, Shiroff et al. (2022, p. 49) concluded that:

> Reintegration into civilian life by veterans' post deployment is incredibly challenging. Veterans, by nature of their culture and the stigma attached to mental health disorders such as PTSD and TBI, oftentimes do not seek professional help. This qualitative research supports the use of SDs [Service Dogs] who are trained to mitigate the negative effects of PTSD and TBI in veterans post deployment regardless of having a concomitant physical disability. As noted by one study participant: "He's the reason I am still alive."

2.1.2 Family Members of Veterans

An examination of the citations retrieved from the PubMed search yielded three studies in which the impact of a service dog for PTSD from the perspective of the partners of veterans who used these animals was documented (McCall et al., 2020; Nieforth et al., 2022a, 2022b).

PTSD can have a detrimental impact on family relationships. However, there are studies about the impact that psychiatric service dogs have on the partners of veterans. To address this limitation, in McCall et al.'s (2020) mixed-methods study 60 veteran–partner pairs were either paired with a service dog (service dog group; *n*

= 37) or waited for a placement (waitlist group; $n = 23$). The partners in the service dog group reported greater levels of resilience and companionship, and lower levels of anger, social isolation, and work impairment compared to those in the control group. Additionally, the data from the survey showed that service dogs provided more benefits than challenges, including improvements in veteran functioning, family relationships, and partners' quality of life. While these findings are preliminary, they suggest that service dogs may offer positive experiences for certain veteran families.

Nieforth et al. (2022b) evaluated the impact of PTSD service dogs on spouses and families of United States military veterans with assessments at baseline and at three months follow-up. A total of 88 veteran spouses completed a survey at baseline and three months later. The 88 veteran spouses were divided into an intervention group that received a service dog shortly after baseline ($n = 48$) and a waitlist control group ($n = 40$). The results showed that spouses with service dogs in their homes experienced significantly lower caregiver satisfaction, greater caregiver burden, and more participation in life activities in comparison to those on the waitlist. These findings suggest that while service dogs may improve the wellbeing of veterans with PTSD, partners or children of veterans may not experience the same benefits. Considering these findings, clinicians should consider family-focused approaches when interacting with a service dog.

Nieforth et al. (2022a) examined the daily emotional experiences of partners of veterans who had been allocated service dogs for their PTSD. As a part of a larger clinical study, a group of 87 partners of post-9/11 veterans with PTSD were selected from a non-profit organisation that provided service dogs. They took part in an ecological momentary assessment program. The participants included partners of veterans who received a PTSD service dog after the baseline (i.e., treatment group; $n = 48$) and partners of veterans who were on the waitlist for a service dog (i.e., control group; $n = 39$). Data were collected twice daily for two weeks at baseline and again at a three-month follow-up, resulting in approximately 56 assessments per participant (28 at baseline, 28 at follow-up). On average, participants completed 84% of questionnaires at baseline and 86% at follow-up. The findings indicated that partners of veterans with service dogs reported significantly higher levels of positive emotions compared to partners in the control group three months after the initial assessment. Their study provides quantitative evidence indicating that partners who lived with a PTSD service dog reported greater levels of positive emotions compared to those partners who were on the waitlist. The influence of service dogs may extend beyond veterans to impact their partners, given the positive impact of emotions on wellbeing and coping (Nieforth et al., 2022a).

2.1.3 Elderly

Although assistance dogs and the therapeutic benefits they bring has been a popular topic for research, there have been few studies that have examined their benefits for older adults. From the PubMed search one study was identified that examined the therapeutic benefits that assistance dogs can provide elderly people (Salmon & Pachana, 2022). Salmon and Pachana (2022) assessed the therapeutic benefits of assistance dogs on the practical, mental, physical, and social wellbeing of older adults. Their systematic review also focused on older adults with disabilities who received support from a guide, hearing, or other types of assistance dog. Out of 2,951 retrieved studies, 256 were assessed for eligibility, and 28 were included in their review. The studies that they examined showed that all types of assistance dogs demonstrated benefits in all assessed domains. However, there were identified disadvantages and barriers to service dog acquisition. Their study suggests that obtaining an assistance dog could have positive clinical impacts, including improved mental health and everyday functioning. Despite these benefits, Salmon and Pachana (2022, p. 23) claimed that:

> … this review has highlighted several notable gaps within the literature, which should be addressed in future research. First, despite assistance-animals receiving increased attention, there is a lack of studies that are methodologically robust. Second, there is a lack of assistance dog studies that focus exclusively on older adults. Given that some studies may be confounded by younger people being more likely to acquire an assistance dog, coupled with the increased needs of older adults with age-related health decline, this is a key area to be addressed.

2.1.4 People with Disabilities

An examination of the citations retrieved from the PubMed search revealed six studies in which the impact of assistance dogs on people with disabilities was examined (Futeran et al., 2022; Grandgeorge et al., 2023; Gravrok et al., 2020; Rodriguez et al., 2020a, 2020b; Singleton, 2023). To better understand the outcome of research about assistance dogs, Futeran et al. (2022) collected potentially relevant citations from six databases and summarised the results in accordance with the domains from the *International Classification of Functioning, Disability and Health* (ICF) framework. The results of their review indicated that assistance dogs can help people with physical disabilities, mental illness, autism, and chronic conditions requiring alertness, such as epilepsy and diabetes. Using the ICF framework, the reviewed research also suggested that assistance dogs can have a positive impact on participation in numerous aspects of life.

Despite companion dogs being more affordable and easier to obtain, no studies have compared their effectiveness with improving the handler's quality of life compared to assistance dogs. To address this gap, Gravrok et al. (2020) developed and distributed among assistance dog organisations a survey for participants that was based on the Thriving Through Relationships theory. Participants who completed the survey were divided into three groups:

- People with disabilities who had an assistance dog ($n = 165$),
- People without disabilities who had a companion dog ($n = 198$), and
- People with disabilities who had a companion dog ($n = 249$).

The perceived level of support differed significantly between the groups, with assistance dog owners reporting significantly greater levels of support than companion dog owners, regardless of disability status. Compared to companion dogs, assistance dogs were also perceived to offer more support in nine out of ten indicators of the Thriving Through Relationships theory. In essence, assistance dogs were perceived to offer support that can enhance the ability of people with disabilities to thrive. Additionally, for people with disabilities assistance dogs may provide greater support than companion dogs, making them worth the additional time and financial cost. Their study suggests that assistance dogs could also aid in rehabilitation by improving coping skills, particularly during challenging times. Finally, it is also important to note that assistance dogs and companion dogs are not interchangeable in terms of support for people with disabilities (Gravrok et al., 2020).

The aim of Grandgeorge et al.'s (2023) study was to explore the effect of the COVID-19 lockdown on the relationship between people with disabilities and their service dogs. They hypothesised that the lockdown, which reduced social contact and altered human relationships, would have an impact on the relationship between people with disabilities and their service dogs. To investigate this hypothesis, an online survey was completed by 70 participants during the first COVID-19 lockdown in France. The results collected showed that compared to other times during the COVID-19 lockdown, scores from the *Perceived Emotional Closeness and Perceived Costs* subscales were significantly greater while scores for the *Dog-Owner Interaction* subscales were significantly less. These findings suggest that service dogs, like other pets, during the COVID-19 lockdown were a source of emotional support for their owners.

Rodriguez et al. (2020a) assessed the impact that service dogs had on the psychosocial wellbeing and overall health among people with physical disabilities or chronic conditions. In their study, 154 individuals took part in a cross-sectional survey, consisting of 97 participants already partnered with a mobility or medical service dog and 57 participants awaiting placement on a service dog waitlist. Using hierarchical regression analysis, they assessed the impact of owning a service dog on standardised assessments of psychosocial health, including the *Pediatric Quality of Life Inventory*. Additionally, measures such as anger, companionship, and sleep disturbance were evaluated using the *Patient Reported Outcome Measurement Information System*. For participants with a service dog, the *Monash Dog–Owner Relationship Scale* was utilised to quantify the strength of the human–animal bond. Based on the data collected, they concluded that:

> In this study, the provision of a medical or mobility service dog was associated with better psychosocial health among a large, heterogeneous sample of individuals with disabilities and chronic conditions. Specifically, having a service dog was significantly associated with higher social, emotional, and work/school functioning, but was not significantly associated with anger, companionship, or sleep disturbance. These effects were independent of variation due to age, sex, disability impairment and progressiveness, and having a pet dog in the home. Overall, the results of this study suggest that in addition to the functional benefits of a service dog such as mobility assistance, medical alert, and seizure response, their placement may also afford measurable psychosocial benefits to the daily lives of individuals with physical disabilities or chronic conditions. (Rodriguez et al., 2020a, pp. 1356–1357)

Rodriguez et al. (2020b) conducted a qualitative study to compare the anticipated expectations and real-life experiences associated with living alongside a mobility or medical service dog among people with physical disabilities or chronic conditions. They distributed an open-ended survey to 64 participants who were already living with a service dog and 27 participants on a waitlist to receive a service dog. Qualitative content analysis was applied to the collected data to identify and categorise recurring themes and sub-themes within the participants' responses. Their analysis revealed 101 codes that were placed into the following categories: Physical Benefits, Psychosocial Benefits, and Drawbacks associated with owning a service dog. Psychosocial benefits encompassed aspects like the bond between humans and animals, emotional wellbeing, improvements in quality of life, and social advantages. Drawbacks involved responsibilities related to service dog care, challenges concerning public access and education, adjustments in daily routines, and issues with dog behaviour. Notably, those awaiting a service dog appeared more inclined to expect physical advantages, whereas those already paired with a service dog predominantly highlighted the psychosocial benefits. Additionally, the research findings suggest that certain drawbacks, including experiencing discrimination in public settings, were unforeseen by those on the waitlist. Based on these results, Rodriguez et al. (2020b, p. 508) concluded that:

> this study compared the expectations and experiences of both future and current mobility and medical service dog owners to describe the benefits and drawbacks to service dog ownership. Results suggest that in combination with the medical and physical benefits the service dog is trained to provide, those with a service dog experience substantial psychosocial benefits from their service dog's assistance and companionship to a degree that may be unanticipated by future service dog owners. The study's findings provide evidence to suggest that the social, emotional, and quality of life benefits from a service dog's assistance and companionship are an important aspect of the service dog–owner relationship. Further, the drawbacks of having a service dog, specifically those that involve the service dog's behaviour and public access and education, are important considerations to prepare those anticipating the addition of a service dog in their lives.

In the United States of America, over 61 million people have disabilities, yet less than one per cent are paired with service dogs. Such dogs are specifically trained to execute tasks related to a disability, aiding individuals and promoting their self-reliance. They also offer additional benefits. Singleton's (2023) research aimed to provide empirical data on the advantages of being matched with a service dog. Out of 204 respondents paired with service dogs, demographic information and survey responses were collected, focusing on the benefits they derive from this partnership. The overwhelming consensus among participants indicated significant positive effects, including emotional connection, increased community engagement, enhanced physical activity, improved psychological wellbeing, elevated quality of life, reduced reliance on prescribed medications, and a decrease in required assistance hours (see Table 2.3). Notably, these benefits extend beyond addressing their primary disability needs. These results show that service dogs have the potential to benefit people with disabilities by addressing primary and ancillary needs that foster independence. However, there is a need for stronger evidence to provide more tangible support for people seeking service dog partnerships.

Table 2.3 Benefits of being teamed with a service dog

Question[a]	Strongly Agree (%)	Somewhat Agree (%)	Somewhat Disagree (%)	Strongly Disagree (%)
1. My service dog helps to improve my emotional connections to others	79	17	2	1
2. My service dog helps me to participate in my community	73	24	2	1
3. My serviced dog helps me to be physically active	75	20	2	1
4. My service dog helps me with my psychological wellbeing	85	13	2	0.49
5. My service dog helps me to have a good quality of life	84	13	1	6
6. Having a service dog has helped my health care provider to decrease my mediations	48	31	15	6
7. Having a service dog has helped to decrease the assistance hours, paid and/ or unpaid hours, for care I receive to support my needs	54	30	9	6

Note [a]Across all 7 questions, there was a 1% no response rate
Source Singleton (2023, p. 7)

2.1.5 People with Dementia

Three studies about the potential benefits that people with dementia can obtain from service dogs were identified from the citations generated from the PubMed search (Marks & McVilly, 2020, 2023; Vincent et al., 2023). Marks and McVilly's (2020) systematic review examined the effectiveness of trained assistance dogs in supporting people with dementia. They examined peer-reviewed articles from multiple databases (i.e., SCOPUS, Web of Science, and Google Scholar), and screened reference lists to identify other studies for inclusion. The 24 studies examined reported findings on the potential positive effects of dog-assisted interventions in relation to mood, prosocial behaviours, activities of daily living, quality of life, cognitive impairment, and symptoms specific to dementia. However, the studies varied in quality and no specific studies were found about the benefits of assistance dogs for those with younger onset dementia (YOD). Their review suggests that more research is needed, particularly with larger samples and designs incorporating control groups. Mixed-methods could be employed to allow for the triangulation of qualitative and quantitative data. Additionally, studies need to be concluded over time because conditions like dementia, and other deteriorating conditions, change over time. Finally, their review also suggests that the effects of dog-assisted interventions on the wider family should be considered since family members are often influential in the lives of those with dementia (Marks & McVilly, 2020).

There is a growing body of evidence supporting the benefits of trained assistance dogs for promoting the health, wellbeing, and quality of life of people with various disabilities, including those with dementia. However, little is known about the experiences of people with YOD and their family. Marks and McVilly's (2023) study was part of a larger research project involving 14 people with YOD who were matched with trained assistance dogs over a two-year period. Their study examined the experiences of ten family carers who were interviewed on multiple occasions to investigate their experiences with an assistance dog. Their results showed that the family carers had a range of experiences, both positive and challenging. Their findings fell into three main categories, which were: the human–animal bond, relationship dynamics, and responsibility for caring. They concluded that while trained assistance dogs can play a crucial role in promoting the health and wellbeing of people with YOD and their family, concerns were raised regarding the financial resources needed to support an assistance dog (Marks & McVilly, 2023).

Vincent et al. (2023) compared the effectiveness of canine assistance for family caregivers and people with dementia in three scenarios caregiver and person with mild to moderate dementia paired with either (1) a neuro service dog (NSD), (2) a companion dog, or (3) no dog. The study encompassed five caregivers with an NSD, 28 caregivers with a companion dog, and 23 caregivers without a dog. The examination of roles and functions of the dog revealed that *'Socialization'* and *'Assistance with direction'* were the most addressed roles for dyads with an NSD. Conversely, for dyads with a companion dog or no dog, *'Engagement and finding meaning in life'* and *'Physical activity involving the dog'* were the predominant roles discussed. The role related to *'Sleep or waking up'* was the least discussed across all three cases. Regarding home care support, the presence of an NSD exhibited more positive impacts on both people with dementia and their caregivers compared to the presence of a companion dog. Furthermore, people with dementia accompanied by an NSD accessed more indoor and outdoor public sites compared to those with a companion dog. Lastly, dyads with a dog were more frequently engaged in informal social activities compared to those without a dog. Finally, they proposed a conceptual framework about the usability of an NSD for caregivers living with someone with dementia (see Fig. 2.1).

2.1.6 People with Mental Health Disorders

From the citations retrieved from the PubMed search one study was identified in which the therapeutic benefits of assistance dogs for people with mental health disorders were measured (Lloyd et al., 2019). Lloyd et al. (2019) studied a population of people with mental health disorders who owned psychiatric assistance dogs (PADs). Their sample was composed of 199 PAD owners in Australia who were registered with the charity *mindDOG*. They reported that PAD owners had different mental health diagnoses and that their dogs performed different tasks to support them in daily life. Tasks that PADs performed included reduction of anxiety through tactile

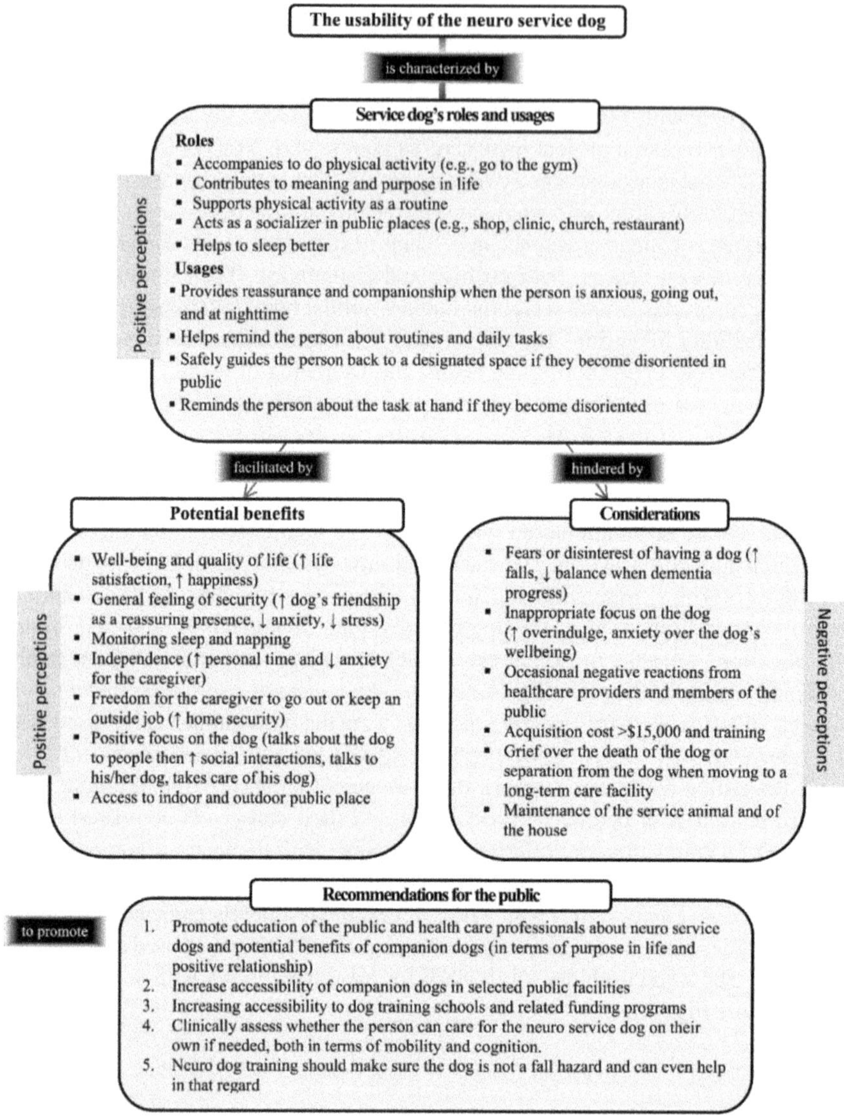

Fig. 2.1 Usability of the neuro service dog for the caregiver living with a person with dementia: a proposed conceptual framework. *Note* ↑ increase or improve; ↓ decrease or reduce. *Source* Vincent et al. (2023, p. 1855)

stimulation, nudging/pawing to bring back to the present, interrupting undesirable behaviour, constant body contact, deep pressure stimulation, and blocking contact from other people (see Fig. 2.2). Their study highlights the importance of understanding this population and the person–dog relationship to inform the appropriate

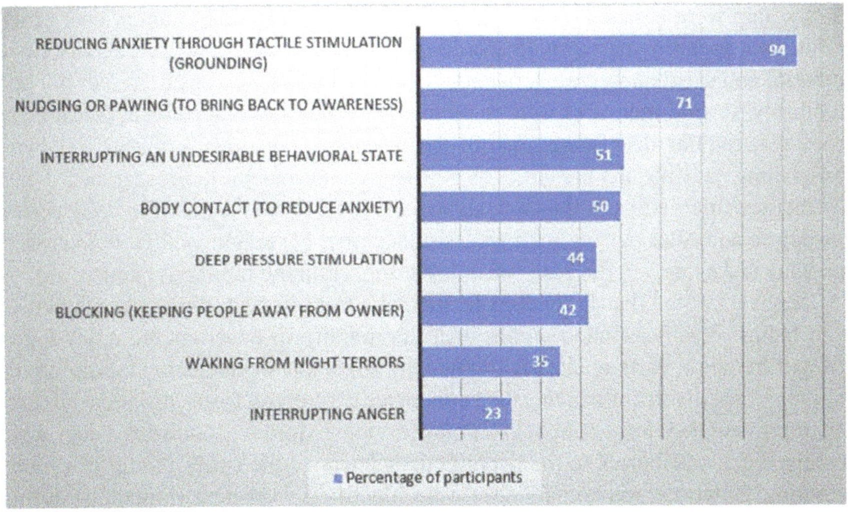

Fig. 2.2 Tasks performed by the psychiatric assistance dogs for the participants. *Source* Lloyd et al. (2019, p. 4)

choice, training, and use of PADs for people living with mental health problems (Lloyd et al., 2019).

2.1.7 *Autistic Children*

Five studies were identified from the citations collected from the PubMed search that described the therapeutic benefits that assistance dogs give autistic children (Agnew et al., 2023; Dollion et al., 2021, 2022; Leung et al., 2022; Tseng, 2023). The results of these studies are now presented.

Autism is a developmental condition marked by alterations in social interaction, communication, and behaviour. Dogs trained for assistance have shown the potential to aid children with autism in participating in daily activities. Despite a growing number of children being paired with these dogs, there is a scarcity of research about how these assistance dogs specifically influence the involvement of children with autism and their families in daily routines. More comprehensive research is necessary to grasp fully the effects and significance of this support system, particularly within Australia. To address this gap, Agnew et al. (2023) investigated the firsthand experiences shared by caregivers regarding the impact of an assistance dog on the involvement of children with autism in daily activities, as well as the effects on their families' engagement.

Employing a qualitative methodology, Agnew et al. conducted semi-structured interviews with six caregivers responsible for seven children diagnosed with autism, all of whom were assisted by an individual assistance dog. These interviews varied in duration, spanning between 45 and 60 min each. The interviews were transcribed verbatim and subsequently underwent a thematic analysis. To ensure reliability and credibility, several measures were implemented, including independent recruitment processes, regular discussions within the research team, member checking with participants, and the maintenance of a reflective journal by the researcher. Three key themes emerged from the analysis: (1) the level of involvement in daily activities before and after pairing with an assistance dog, (2) heightened participation in everyday tasks, and (3) the assistance dog's impact on the family dynamic.

Caregivers noted that these dogs facilitated a transition for children with autism from being socially isolated within their community to experiencing a newfound sense of freedom. Participants highlighted the dog's role in enhancing the children's abilities by positively influencing their adherence to routines, fostering independence, and improving their engagement in therapy sessions. Moreover, assistance dogs were perceived as contributors to the overall engagement of the entire family in various activities. However, some challenges were identified, including difficulties during the introduction of the assistance dog to the family, financial burdens related to the maintenance of the animal, time commitments, issues concerning public access rights, and the limited availability of government funding to support this assistance (Agnew et al., 2023).

The use of assistance dogs has been shown to be effective in improving the quality of life and prompting social and community participation for autistics. Leung et al. (2022) evaluated the outcomes of assistance dogs on the quality of life, independence, and participation of families with an autistic child. They conducted a cross-section comparative study, using various measures to evaluate adaptive skills, behaviour, social difficulties, daily functioning, and family quality of life. Six families who had an Autism Assistance Dog (AAD) placed with them were compared to 12 families on the waiting list for an AAD. Their study showed that there were no significant differences between the two groups, but there were trends suggesting that AADs can increase desired social behaviours, decrease the severity of autistic symptoms, and improve family wellbeing. Additionally, families who were partnered with an AAD for longer showed more positive outcomes. The findings of their study contribute to the growing evidence about the benefits that AADs give autistic children.

Recognising and interpreting facial expressions is crucial for social interaction in humans. Research has indicated that autistics encounter difficulties deciphering facial expressions, which may be linked to altered strategies in visually scanning expressive faces. Although previous studies have highlighted the positive effects of pet and service dogs on the social skills and psychological development of autistic children, there are no studies about whether these benefits extend to the processing of facial expressions. In response, Dollion et al. (2022) investigated if owning a service dog influenced the facial expression processing skills of autistic children. Two groups of 15 autistic children, one group with and one group without a service dog, were assessed by a computer-based facial expression recognition task, while their ocular movements were recorded using an eye-tracking device. While the accuracy and reaction time of both groups did not differ significantly, autistic children who owned a service dog demonstrated a reduced focus on irrelevant areas of the face during facial expression processing. They also exhibited more distinctive scanning of specific facial features corresponding to the expressed emotion (i.e., more time spent on the mouth for joy than for anger, and vice versa for the eyes area). The outcomes of their study suggest that owning a service dog and regularly interacting with it may facilitate the development of targeted visual exploration techniques for processing human facial expressions.

Dollion et al. (2021) conducted two experiments that were focused on the relationship between the visual attention of autistic children and their behaviours during their first interaction with a service dog. For their first experiment the researchers conducted video behavioural analyses of 16 autistic children who interacted with a service dog. Their second experiment was exploratory and involved six children. The researchers used the same behavioural approach as in the first experiment, but they also included eye-tracking data. Their experiments found that the more autistic children looked at both their parent and the evaluator, instead of inanimate items, the more they interacted with the service dog. These two experiments shed light on how visual attention may impact the interaction between autistic children and service dogs and may inform future training and placement of service dogs for autistic children (Dollion et al., 2021).

Tseng (2023) used a within-subject, repeated-measure design to assess changes in psychological and bio-behavioural outcomes before and after families received a trained AAD. Their study included data from 11 trails (i.e., parent/handler-dog-child), and was the first to assess changes in a biomarker for chronic stress in both autistic children and their parents. Overall, their study found significantly positive effects of AADs on both psychological and bio-behavioural outcomes. Specifically, the children showed improvements in social interaction and emotional regulation, while the parents reported decreased stress and improved quality of life. They also reported a decrease in cortisol levels, a biomarker for chronic stress, in both the children and their parents after introducing ADDs. These findings provide empirical support for the use of AADs as a complementary intervention for autistic children and their families.

2.2 Documented Experiences About Parents Using an Assistance or Service Dog for Their Children

Four studies were discovered from the PubMed search that contained descriptions about the experiences that parents had regarding their child with a disability using a dog. Two studies described such experiences from the perspective of parents raising autistic children (Appleby et al., 2022; Hellings et al., 2022). The other two studies described such experiences from the perspective of parents who were raising children with different disabilities (Bibbo et al., 2019; Lindsay & Thiyagarajah, 2021). An overview and the results of these four studies are documented below.

Assistance dogs have been found to provide safety and decrease stress and isolation for families of autistic children. However, little is known about parents' experiences of owning an AAD. To address this gap in the literature, Appleby et al. (2022) conducted a mixed-methods study using a qualitative descriptive design and occupational mapping. Eight families were recruited from an Australian AAD program and they participated in semi-structured in-depth interviews, which were thematically analysed. Mobility in the community before and after introducing the AAD was measured using occupational mapping, where families plotted on Google Maps the places that they frequented before and after placement of their dog. Results showed that families with an AAD experienced expanded mobility for the child, as the dog provided increased freedom and safety, decreased isolation, and served as a calming and sensory tool. These results provide support for funding and increased awareness of AAD programs. However, more longitudinal studies are needed to examine the long-term impact of AADs on their child and family.

According to Hellings et al. (2022) there has been no exploration of the actual experiences of families who have recently acquired assistance animals. Their research aimed to uncover the expectations, benefits, and challenges of owning assistance animals for families with autistic children. Semi-structured interviews and photovoice were used to gather data from four mothers, both before the placement of the assistance animals and six months after ownership. The results revealed that owning assistance animals improved the autistic children's self-regulation and socialisation and led to an increased engagement in everyday activities. Additionally, assistance animals contributed to greater family involvement in outings and other events. Nevertheless, some difficulties were encountered during the adjustment period and the public's lack of knowledge regarding autism assistance animals was a challenge.

Not much is known about the impact that service dogs have on the family members of people with chronic illnesses. Bibbo et al. (2019) addressed this gap by measuring the impact of service dogs on the functioning of family members. Data were collected through an online, telephone, or mail-based self-reported survey. Participants were recruited from *Canine Assistants*; a national service dog provider. The participants were caregivers or spouses of people with disabilities or illnesses who either had a service dog ($n = 51$) or were on a waitlist to receive one ($n = 73$). The final survey included 50 family members (46 parents or caregivers and 4 spouses or partners) living with a service dog and 76 family members (68 parents or caregivers and 8 spouses or partners) who had a family member who was waiting to receive a service dog. They reported that interacting with a service dog contributed to a reduction in health-related concerns, improved overall psychosocial health, enhanced emotional functioning, minimised family impact from the chronic condition, and better emotional health-related quality of life. These results offer evidence suggesting that beyond impacting the recipients themselves, service dogs can influence various facets of family members' psychosocial wellbeing and functionality.

The presence of a service dog has shown potential in enhancing independence and wellbeing for individuals living with disabilities or chronic health conditions. Despite the rising utilisation of service dogs among children and youth, there remains a lack of comprehensive synthesis regarding their overall impact. The objective of Lindsay and Thiyagarajah's (2021) study was to perform a systematic review aimed at evaluating the influence of service dogs on children, youth, and their families. They conducted systematic searches across seven international databases spanning from 1985 to 2020. Their review encompassed 29 studies involving 1,121 children, youth, or their parents representing them across six diverse countries, spanning a 32-year period. They reported that 23 out of the 29 studies discovered described improvements in at least one of the following domains: physical health (e.g., diabetes management, seizure control, mobility), psychological wellbeing (e.g., quality of life, safety, behaviour, stress, anxiety, self-confidence, and independence), social adjustment (e.g., social interactions, school, and work), and the bond between the dog and owner. They concluded that while their findings highlight the potential advantages that service dogs provide for children, youth, and their families, it is imperative to conduct more research employing more robust study designs.

2.3 Views of Professionals About the Usage of Assistance or Service Dogs

An examination of the citations retrieved from the PubMed search revealed three studies about the views of professionals about the usage of assistance or service dogs for people with disabilities (Chan et al., 2022; Iong et al., 2022; Merk et al., 2021). A description of these studies and their findings are presented in this section.

Support dogs perform numerous tasks to help people with disabilities. Occupational therapists hold a pivotal position in evaluating and directing patients towards assistive technology. However, limited information exists regarding Australian occupational therapists understanding of support dogs. To address this lack of knowledge, Chan et al. (2022) created and distributed a nationwide online survey among Australian occupational therapists to uncover their encounters and perspectives regarding support dogs, as well as to gather their suggestions for enhancing their practices.

Chan et al. examined 220 completed surveys and discovered that all respondents expressed recognition of the benefits that assistance dogs offer to clients with disabilities. While more than 60% agreed that assessing or referring clients to support or assistance dogs fell within their professional responsibilities, more than two-thirds had not yet encountered such opportunities due to their lacking relevant training or not having had the chance to engage in this aspect of their practice. Challenges commonly encountered during the referral or assessment process included difficulties in accessing funding, navigating resources, a perceived shortage of both service or assistance dogs, and inconclusive evidence supporting their use. Their findings indicate that while occupational therapists recognise the importance of assistance dogs within their practice, there exists a prevalent lack of practical experience and comprehensive understanding. This finding underscores the critical need for specialised professional development opportunities tailored explicitly for occupational therapists. This need is becoming increasingly significant given the rising visibility and wider range of applications for assistance dogs.

Iong et al. (2022) also aimed to investigate the level of understanding and viewpoints of Australian occupational therapists concerning assistance dogs. They explored their knowledge regarding the National Disability Insurance Scheme (NDIS) funding for animal support and resources that they believed were valuable in facilitating occupational therapy assessments and report writing. The findings from their research underscore the importance of improved information dissemination among occupational therapists concerning diverse categories of assistance dogs and the regulatory framework of NDIS funding. Introducing NDIS reporting templates, offering practical guidelines, and providing resources for professional development—coupled with integrating content into occupational therapy curricula for upcoming therapists—could significantly augment their knowledge base, clinical decision-making, and practice.

Merk et al. (2021) evaluated the familiarity that health professionals had with regulations concerning the American with Disabilities Act (ADA) and their perceptions about workplace protocols and training concerning service dogs. To explore this topic they created a survey that had 24 items. In total, 441 professionals in the healthcare industry from around the United States of America completed the survey. At the time of completing the survey, most respondents worked in a hospital (n = 234, 53.1%) and were employed in a diverse range of occupations, including nursing (n = 155, 35.2%) and medicine (n = 71, 16.1%). Almost three-quarters of respondents (n = 318, 73.1%) were aware that their workplace had a policy about service animals. However, 113 (34.9%) of these respondents claimed that they were not fully versed in the policy and 236 (54.5%) stated that they had not received any training about the topic. Based on these findings Merk et al. (2021, p. 247) concluded:

> Our results suggest that increased familiarity and training leads to higher knowledge about service dogs and ADA policy. Health professionals need additional education on ADA service dog regulations and hospital policy in order to minimize risk and ensure patients with service dogs receive optimal care.

2.4 Conclusion

This chapter presented the literature from the PubMed search about the benefits that people with different disabilities obtained from their interactions with assistance or service dogs. It was revealed that such benefits included increased socialisation, greater independence, quality of life, and an improved sense of security and well-being. In the next chapter, the limitations of the studies described in this chapter are presented.

References

Agnew, Z., Callaway, L., Lalor, A., Peart, A., & Bould, E. (2023). 'Having the dog as part of our family gives us hope': Experiences of the impact of assistance dogs on the occupational engagement of children with autism and their families. *Australian Occupational Therapy Journal*. Advance online publication. https://doi.org/10.1111/1440-1630.12904

Appleby, R., Wright, S., Williams, L., & Stanley, M. (2022). Australian parents' experiences of owning an autism assistance dog. *Health & Social Care in the Community, 30*(6), e4113–e4121. https://doi.org/10.1111/hsc.13805

Bibbo, J., Rodriguez, K. E., & O'Haire, M. E. (2019). Impact of service dogs on family members' psychosocial functioning. *The American Journal of Occupational Therapy: Official Publication of the American Occupational Therapy Association, 73*(3), 7303205120p1–7303205120p11. https://doi.org/10.5014/ajot.2019.031690

Brown, M. (2015). *Examination of veteran experiences with service animals and animal assisted therapy: A case study* (Doctoral dissertation, The Chicago School of Professional Psychology).

Chan, K. W., Young, J., Williams, L. J., & Nottle, C. (2022). Assistance dogs in occupational therapy practice: A survey of Australian occupational therapists' experiences and recommendations. *Australian Occupational Therapy Journal, 69*(2), 129–139. https://doi.org/10.1111/1440-1630.12775

Crowe, T. K., Nguyen, M. T., Tryon, B. G., Barger, S., & Sanchez, V. (2018b). How service dogs enhance veterans' occupational performance in the home: A qualitative perspective. *The Open Journal of Occupational Therapy, 6*(3), 12. https://doi.org/10.15453/2168-6408.1468

Crowe, T. K., Sánchez, V., Howard, A., Western, B., & Barger, S. (2018b). Veterans transitioning from isolation to integration: A look at veteran/service dog partnerships. *Disability and Rehabilitation, 40*(24), 2953–2961. https://doi.org/10.1080/09638288.2017.1363301

Dollion, N., Grandgeorge, M., Saint-Amour, D., Hosein Poitras Loewen, A., François, N., Fontaine, N. M. G., Champagne, N., & Plusquellec, P. (2022). Emotion facial processing in children with autism spectrum disorder: A pilot study of the impact of service dogs. *Frontiers in Psychology, 13*, 869452. https://doi.org/10.3389/fpsyg.2022.869452

Dollion, N., Toutain, M., François, N., Champagne, N., Plusquellec, P., & Grandgeorge, M. (2021). Visual exploration and observation of real-life interactions between children with ASD and service dogs. *Journal of Autism and Developmental Disorders, 51*(11), 3785–3805. https://doi.org/10.1007/s10803-021-05293-1

Floore-Guetschow, L. (2020). *Exploring the effect of service dogs on PTSD symptoms in veterans*. The University of Wisconsin—Milwaukee.

Futeran, N., Mackenzie, L., Wilkes-Gillan, S., & Dickson, C. (2022). Understanding the participation outcomes for persons with disability when partnered with assistance dogs: A scoping review. *Australian Occupational Therapy Journal, 69*(4), 475–492. https://doi.org/10.1111/1440-1630.12801

Galsgaard, A., & Eskelund, K. (2020). An explorative clinical pilot study into the effect of service dogs on chronic posttraumatic stress disorder. *Traumatology, 26*(4), 361. https://doi.org/10.1037/trm0000278

Genbauffe, C. (2020). *Using exposure therapy and service dogs to treat PTSD: Pragmatic case studies*. Rutgers The State University of New Jersey, Graduate School of Applied and Professional Psychology.

Grandgeorge, M., Rochais, C., Auffret, F., & Dollion, N. (2023). Service dogs and persons with disabilities: When COVID-19 lockdown changes their relationship. *Animals: An Open Access Journal from MDPI, 13*(5), 914. https://doi.org/10.3390/ani13050914

Gravrok, J., Howell, T., Bendrups, D., & Bennett, P. (2020). Thriving through relationships: Assistance dogs' and companion dogs' perceived ability to contribute to thriving in individuals with and without a disability. *Disability and Rehabilitation. Assistive Technology, 15*(1), 45–53. https://doi.org/10.1080/17483107.2018.1513574

Hansen, C. (2019). *The impact of service dogs on combat veterans with posttraumatic stress disorder*. Walden University.

Hansen, C., Iannos, M., & Van Hooff, M. (2023). Assistance dogs help reduce mental health symptoms among Australian Defence Force veterans and emergency services personnel: A pilot study. *Psychiatry research, 324*, 115212. https://doi.org/10.1016/j.psychres.2023.115212

Hellings, D., Joosten, A., Hatfield, M., & Netto, J. (2022). Benefits and challenges of assistance dogs for families of children on the autism spectrum: Mothers' perspectives. *Qualitative Health Research, 32*(11), 1648–1656. https://doi.org/10.1177/10497323221111247

Husband, A., Ahmed, A., & Dell, C. A. (2020). An exploratory case study of the impact of psychiatric service dogs on problematic substance use among PTSD-diagnosed veterans. *Journal of Substance Use, 25*(2), 113–117. https://doi.org/10.1080/14659891.2019.1664663

Hyde, J. N. (2015). *Service dogs: An exploratory pilot study of a complementary approach to evidence-based treatment of PTSD in combat veterans of the Iraq and Afghanistan wars* (Doctoral dissertation, Adler School of Professional Psychology).

Iong, K. K., Bould, E., Lalor, A., & Callaway, L. (2022). Australian occupational therapists' knowledge of the purpose, scope, and funding of assistance dogs. *Australian Occupational Therapy Journal, 69*(1), 64–76. https://doi.org/10.1111/1440-1630.12770

Jensen, C. L., Rodriguez, K. E., & O'Haire, M. E. (2021). Service dogs for veterans and military members with posttraumatic stress disorder: Replication with the PTSD checklist for DSM-5. *Journal of Traumatic Stress, 34*, 221–228. https://doi.org/10.1002/jts.22587

Jensen, C. L., Rodriguez, K. E., MacLean, E. L., Abdul Wahab, A. H., Sabbaghi, A., & O'Haire, M. E. (2022). Characterizing veteran and PTSD service dog teams: Exploring potential mechanisms of symptom change and canine predictors of efficacy. *PLoS ONE, 17*(7), e0269186. https://doi.org/10.1371/journal.pone.0269186

Kegel, A. (2016). *Service dogs for the mind: Psychiatric service dogs for the treatment of post-traumatic stress disorder and alcohol use in veterans: A quantitative study*. The Wright Institute.

Kloep, M. L., Hunter, R. H., & Kertz, S. J. (2017). Examining the effects of a novel training program and use of psychiatric service dogs for military-related PTSD and associated symptoms. *The American Journal of Orthopsychiatry, 87*(4), 425–433. https://doi.org/10.1037/ort0000254

Kopicki, A. (2016). *Examining the efficacy of service dogs as an alternative intervention for veterans diagnosed with posttraumatic stress disorder* (Doctoral dissertation, Adler University).

LaFollette, M. R., Rodriguez, K. E., Ogata, N., & O'Haire, M. E. (2019). Military veterans and their PTSD service dogs: Associations between training methods, PTSD severity, dog behavior, and the human-animal bond. *Frontiers in Veterinary Science, 6*, 23. https://doi.org/10.3389/fvets.2019.00023

Leighton, S. C., Nieforth, L. O., & O'Haire, M. E. (2022). Assistance dogs for military veterans with PTSD: A systematic review, meta-analysis, and meta-synthesis. *PLoS ONE, 17*(9), e0274960. https://doi.org/10.1371/journal.pone.0274960

Lessard, G., Gagnon, D. H., Vincent, C., & PTSD-Service Dog Research Team. (2020). Changes in physical activity and sleep among veterans using a service dog as a rehabilitation modality for post-traumatic stress disorder: An open-label single-arm exploratory trial using actigraphy-based measures. *Journal of Psychosocial Rehabilitation and Mental Health, 7*, 243–262. https://doi.org/10.1007/s40737-020-00187-4

Lessard, G., Vincent, C., Gagnon, D. H., Belleville, G., Auger, É., Lavoie, V., Besemann, M., Champagne, N., Dumont, F. & Béland, E. (2018). Psychiatric service dogs as a tertiary prevention modality for veterans living with post-traumatic stress disorder. *Mental Health & Prevention, 10*, 42–49. https://doi.org/10.1016/j.mhp.2018.01.002

Leung, J. Y., Mackenzie, L., & Dickson, C. (2022). Outcomes of assistance dog placement in the home for individuals with autism spectrum disorder and their families: A pilot study. *Australian Occupational Therapy Journal, 69*(1), 50–63. https://doi.org/10.1111/1440-1630.12768

Lindsay, S., & Thiyagarajah, K. (2021). The impact of service dogs on children, youth and their families: A systematic review. *Disability and Health Journal, 14*(3), 101012. https://doi.org/10.1016/j.dhjo.2020.101012

Lloyd, J., Johnston, L., & Lewis, J. (2019). Psychiatric assistance dog use for people living with mental health disorders. *Frontiers in Veterinary Science, 6*, 166. https://doi.org/10.3389/fvets.2019.00166

Marks, G., & McVilly, K. (2020). Trained assistance dogs for people with dementia: A systematic review. *Psychogeriatrics: The Official Journal of the Japanese Psychogeriatric Society, 20*(4), 510–521. https://doi.org/10.1111/psyg.12529

Marks, G., & McVilly, K. R. (2023). Assistance dogs for people with younger (early)-onset dementia: The family carer's experience. *Animals: An Open Access Journal from MDPI, 13*(5), 777. https://doi.org/10.3390/ani13050777

Marston, H. (2015). *An efficacy study regarding the impact of service dogs on the quality of life of combat veterans*. Adler School of Professional Psychology.

McCall, C. E., Rodriguez, K. E., Wadsworth, S. M. M., Meis, L. A., & O'Haire, M. E. (2020). "A part of our family"? Effects of psychiatric service dogs on quality of life and relationship functioning in military-connected couples. *Military Behavioral Health, 8*(4), 410–423. https://doi.org/10.1080/21635781.2020.1825243

McLaughlin, K., & Hamilton, A. L. (2019). Exploring the influence of service dogs on participation in daily occupations by veterans with PTSD: A pilot study. *Australian Occupational Therapy Journal, 66*(5), 648–655. https://doi.org/10.1111/1440-1630.12606

Merk, A., Nelson, E., Provost, A., Rasch, M., Forster, L., Nottingham, K., Simon, J., & Fredricks, T. (2021). A survey on health professionals' understanding of federal protections regarding service dogs in clinical settings. *Journal of Osteopathic Medicine, 121*(3), 247–253. https://doi.org/10.1515/jom-2020-0280

Moore, A. (2014). *Animal-assisted therapy for United States veterans with posttraumatic stress disorder*. The Wright Institute.

Newton, R. (2014). *Exploring the experiences of living with psychiatric service dogs for veterans with posttraumatic stress disorder*. 1557029 MA. Adler School of Professional Psychology.

Nieforth, L. O., Abdul Wahab, A. H., Sabbaghi, A., MacDermid Wadsworth, S., Foti, D., & O'Haire, M. E. (2022a). Quantifying the emotional experiences of partners of veterans with PTSD service dogs using ecological momentary assessment. *Complementary Therapies in Clinical Practice, 48*, 101590. https://doi.org/10.1016/j.ctcp.2022.101590

Nieforth, L. O., Craig, E. A., Behmer, V. A., MacDermid Wadsworth, S., & O'Haire, M. E. (2023). PTSD service dogs foster resilience among veterans and military families. *Current Psychology, 42*(16), 13207–13219. https://doi.org/10.1007/s12144-021-01990-3

Nieforth, L. O., Miller, E. A., MacDermid Wadsworth, S., & O'Haire, M. E. (2022b). Posttraumatic stress disorder service dogs and the wellbeing of veteran families. *European Journal of Psychotraumatology, 13*(1), 2062997. https://doi.org/10.1080/20008198.2022.2062997

Nieforth, L. O., Rodriguez, K. E., & O'Haire, M. E. (2022c). Expectations versus experiences of veterans with posttraumatic stress disorder (PTSD) service dogs: An inductive conventional content analysis. *Psychological Trauma: Theory, Research, Practice and Policy, 14*(3), 347–356. https://doi.org/10.1037/tra0001021

O'Haire, M. E., & Rodriguez, K. E. (2018). Preliminary efficacy of service dogs as a complementary treatment for posttraumatic stress disorder in military members and veterans. *Journal of Consulting and Clinical Psychology, 86*(2), 179–188. https://doi.org/10.1037/ccp0000267

Parenti, L. (2019). *Service dogs for veterans with PTSD: Taxonomy, work stress reduction, and matching*. West Virginia University.

Richerson, J. T., Saunders, G. H., Skelton, K., Abrams, T., Storzbach, D., Fallon, M. T., Biswas, K., Wagner, T. H., Magruder, K. M., Stock, E. M., & Mi, Z. (2020). *A randomized trial of differential effectiveness of service dog pairing to improve quality of life for veterans with PTSD*. Department of Veterans Affairs. https://www.research.va.gov/REPORT-Study-of-Costs-and-Benefits-Associated-with-the-Use-of-Service-Dogs-Monograph1.pdf

Richerson, J. T., Wagner, T. H., Abrams, T., Skelton, K., Biswas, K., Illarmo, S., McSherry, F., Fallon, M. T., Frakt, A., Pizer, S., Magruder, K. M., Groer, S., Dorn, P. A., Huang, G. D., & Stock, E. M. (2023). Therapeutic and economic benefits of service dogs versus emotional support dogs for veterans with PTSD. *Psychiatric Services (Washington, D.C.), 74*(8), 790–800. https://doi.org/10.1176/appi.ps.20220138

Rodriguez, K. E., Anderson, L. M., Ott, C. A., & O'Haire, M. E. (2021). The effect of a PTSD service dog on military veterans' medication regimens: A cross-sectional pilot study. *Anthrozoos, 34*(3), 393–406. https://doi.org/10.1080/08927936.2021.1898219

Rodriguez, K. E., Bibbo, J., & O'Haire, M. E. (2020a). The effects of service dogs on psychosocial health and wellbeing for individuals with physical disabilities or chronic conditions. *Disability and Rehabilitation, 42*(10), 1350–1358. https://doi.org/10.1080/09638288.2018.1524520

Rodriguez, K. E., Bibbo, J., Verdon, S., & O'Haire, M. E. (2020b). Mobility and medical service dogs: A qualitative analysis of expectations and experiences. *Disability and Rehabilitation. Assistive Technology, 15*(5), 499–509. https://doi.org/10.1080/17483107.2019.1587015

Rodriguez, K. E., Bryce, C. I., Granger, D. A., & O'Haire, M. E. (2018). The effect of a service dog on salivary cortisol awakening response in a military population with posttraumatic stress disorder (PTSD). *Psychoneuroendocrinology, 98*, 202–210. https://doi.org/10.1016/j.psyneuen.2018.04.026

Rodriguez, K. E., LaFollette, M. R., Hediger, K., Ogata, N., & O'Haire, M. E. (2020c). Defining the PTSD service dog intervention: Perceived importance, usage, and symptom specificity of psychiatric service dogs for military veterans. *Frontiers in Psychology, 11*, 1638. https://doi.org/10.3389/fpsyg.2020.01638

Salmon, A. J., & Pachana, N. A. (2022). A systematic review of the effect of assistance dog ownership on practical support, health, and wellbeing: Implications for older adults. *Clinical Gerontologist, 46*(5), 669–694. https://doi.org/10.1080/07317115.2022.2100728

Scotland-Coogan, D. (2019a). Anxiety symptoms and sleep disturbance in veterans with posttraumatic stress disorder: The impact of receiving and training a service dog. *The Qualitative Report, 24*(10), 2655–2674.

Scotland-Coogan, D. (2019b). Relationships, socialization and combat veterans: The impact of receiving and training a service dog. *The Qualitative Report, 24*(8), 1897–1914.

Sherman, M., Hutchinson, A. D., Bowen, H., Iannos, M., & Van Hooff, M. (2023). Effectiveness of operation K9 assistance dogs on suicidality in Australian veterans with PTSD: A 12-month mixed-methods follow-up study. *International Journal of Environmental Research and Public Health, 20*(4), 3607. https://doi.org/10.3390/ijerph20043607

Shiroff, J. J., Gray, K., Santulli, G. M., DiDonato, S., Kelly, P. J., & Fulford, J. O. (2022). A qualitative exploration of the use of service dogs in veterans with post traumatic stress disorder and traumatic brain injury. *Psychiatric Research and Clinical Practice, 5*(2), 40–50. https://doi.org/10.1176/appi.prcp.20220029

Singleton, J. K. (2023). Benefits of being teamed with a service dog for individuals living with visible and invisible disabilities. *Healthcare (Basel, Switzerland), 11*(22), 2987. https://doi.org/10.3390/healthcare11222987

Tilvaldiev, E. (2019). *Future standards for psychiatric service dogs incorporated by veterans who suffer from posttraumatic stress disorder*. The University of the Rockies.

Tseng, A. (2023). Brief report: Above and beyond safety: Psychosocial and biobehavioral impact of autism-assistance dogs on autistic children and their families. *Journal of Autism and Developmental Disorders, 53*(1), 468–483. https://doi.org/10.1007/s10803-021-05410-0

van Houtert, E. A. E., Endenburg, N., Rodenburg, T. B., & Vermetten, E. (2021). Do service dogs for veterans with PTSD mount a cortisol response in response to training? *Animals: An Open Access Journal from MDPI, 11*(3), 650. https://doi.org/10.3390/ani11030650

van Houtert, E. A. E., Rodenburg, T. B., Vermetten, E., & Endenburg, N. (2022). The impact of service dogs on military veterans and (Ex) first aid responders with post-traumatic stress disorder. *Frontiers in Psychiatry, 13*, 834291. https://doi.org/10.3389/fpsyt.2022.834291

Vincent, C., Belleville, G., Gagnon, D. H., Auger, É., Lavoie, V., Besemann, M., & Dumont, F. (2017a). A logic model as the sequence of needs and experience that lead PTSD patients to seek a service dog and concerns related to it: A stakeholders' perspective. *International Journal of Neurorehabil, 4*(268), 2376–281.

Vincent, C., Belleville, G., Gagnon, D. H., Dumont, F., Auger, E., Lavoie, V., Besemann, M., Champagne, N., & Lessart, G. (2017b). Effectiveness of service dogs for veterans with PTSD: Preliminary outcomes. *Studies in Health Technology and Informatics, 242*, 130–136.

Vincent, C., Dumont, F. S., Rivard, A., Rogers, M., Brémault-Phillips, S., Brown, C., & Achou, B. (2023). Roles and usages of neuro service dogs for caregivers living at home with persons with dementia: An exploratory comparative case study. *Dementia (London, England), 22*(8), 1833–1861. https://doi.org/10.1177/14713012231204646

Whitworth, J. D., Scotland-Coogan, D., & Wharton, T. (2019). Service dog training programs for veterans with PTSD: Results of a pilot controlled study. *Social Work in Health Care, 58*(4), 412–430. https://doi.org/10.1080/00981389.2019.1580238

Whitworth, J., O'Brien, C., Wharton, T., & Scotland-Coogan, D. (2020). Understanding partner perceptions of a service dog training program for veterans with PTSD: Building a bridge to trauma resiliency. *Social Work in Mental Health, 18*(6), 604–622. https://doi.org/10.1080/15332985.2020.1806181

Williamson, L., Dell, C. A., Osgood, N., Charlmers, D., Lohnes, C., Carleton, R. N., & Asmundson, G. (2021). Examining changes in posttraumatic stress disorder symptoms and substance use among a sample of Canadian veterans working with service dogs: An exploratory patient-oriented longitudinal study. *Journal of Veteran Studies, 7*(1), 1–13. https://doi.org/10.21061/jvs.v7i1.194

Woodward, S. H., Jamison, A. L., Gala, S., Lawlor, C., Villasenor, D., Tamayo, G., & Puckett, M. (2021). Tracking positive and negative affect in PTSD inpatients during a service dog intervention. *Journal of Consulting and Clinical Psychology, 89*(6), 551–562. https://doi.org/10.1037/ccp0000572

Yarborough, B. J. H., Owen-Smith, A. A., Stumbo, S. P., Yarborough, M. T., Perrin, N. A., & Green, C. A. (2017). An observational study of service dogs for veterans with posttraumatic stress disorder. *Psychiatric Services (Washington, D.C.), 68*(7), 730–734. https://doi.org/10.1176/appi.ps.201500383

Yarborough, B. J. H., Stumbo, S. P., Yarborough, M. T., Owen-Smith, A., & Green, C. A. (2018). Benefits and challenges of using service dogs for veterans with posttraumatic stress disorder. *Psychiatric Rehabilitation Journal, 41*(2), 118–124. https://doi.org/10.1037/prj0000294

Chapter 3
Limitations of Current Studies

3.1 Limitations in the Reviewed Literature About Assistance or Service Dogs

3.1.1 Military Veterans

The primary goal of Hansen et al.'s (2023) pilot study was to assess the efficacy of two specialised Australian assistance dog programs in alleviating Post Traumatic Stress Disorder (PTSD) and mental health symptoms among veterans over the course of one year. Despite its contribution to knowledge, they acknowledged that their study had two limitations. First, there was no control group that received a randomised treatment-as-usual process. To compensate for this limitation, they analysed a subset of participants who underwent assessments while on the waitlist. Second, they speculated that decreases in reported symptoms by the participants during the intervention could be because participants became more accustomed to the assessment tools through repeated use.

Jensen et al. (2022) conducted a longitudinal study that involved 82 post-9/11 military members or veterans and their PTSD service dogs. Their study had three main objectives:

1. To examine the characteristics of the service dogs as potential indicators of effectiveness,
2. To evaluate both dog and human traits as potential factors affecting the bond between veterans and their dogs, and
3. To investigate potential mechanisms contributing to mental health outcomes.

Despite obtaining data that answered these three objectives, they did admit that their study had two limitations. First, while self-reporting can be extremely useful for conveying a participant's personal thoughts and experiences, such as their mental health status, it is worth noting that such insights could have been influenced by

G. Bennett and E. Goodall, *The Role That Assistance Dogs Play in Supporting People with Disabilities*, SpringerBriefs in Modern Perspectives on Disability Research,
https://doi.org/10.1007/978-981-97-1492-6_3

factors like social desirability, participant expectations, and memory recall bias. Second, they acknowledged that their study's sample size was relatively small and drawn from a diverse population, which could have hampered the generalisability of the findings. Adding to this limitation is that the authors recruited participants exclusively from a single service dog provider.

Jensen et al. (2021) used the PTSD Checklist (PCL) based on the fifth edition of the *Diagnostic and Statistical Manual of Mental Disorders* to evaluate the clinical benefits of service dogs on PTSD symptom severity among veterans and military members. Although their study contributed to knowledge it does have two limitations. First, they acknowledged that the occurrence of self-selection/enrolment bias in the sample, where participants had already applied for and been accepted into a single service dog program, restricted the study's applicability to only those who expressed an interest in receiving a service dog and who met the organisation's criteria. Their study's generalisability is further constrained by the characteristics of the sample, including an over-representation of male-identifying participants. Second, they explained that there were three pieces of data that were missing during the data collection phase of the study, potentially limiting their study's interpretations. These omissions were data on recent or ongoing PTSD treatments, the severity of PTSD symptoms prior to receiving a service dog, and details regarding the race and ethnicity of the participants.

LaFollette et al. (2019) investigated the connections between training methods, the severity of PTSD symptoms, the behaviour of the service dog, and the bond between military veterans and their service dogs in a population of veterans dealing with PTSD. While they formulated conclusions about all these factors they did acknowledge that their study had two shortcomings that could have inhibited the interpretation of the results. First, their survey assessed veterans receiving service dogs from a single service dog provider. This focus may have concealed additional relationships that could have been discovered if data from multiple providers were examined. However, it is worth mentioning that they did sample participants from one of the largest providers of PTSD service dogs, that catered to a nationally representative sample of veterans. Consequently, the findings may still hold relevance for a broader population. Second, their survey captured indirect behavioural assessments of service dogs reported by their handlers, which introduces the potential for social desirability bias. The accuracy of their findings could have been improved if they had collected and analysed objective behavioural observations, whether through assessing video recordings along with an assessment of the handlers' overall training philosophies.

Leighton et al. (2022) conducted a systematic review of the literature about the benefits of psychiatric assistance dogs for military veterans with PTSD. They summarised the characteristics of these studies, assessed the quality of the existing evidence, and summarised the outcomes of these studies. While they made a concerted effort to encompass a broad range of studies by searching across 11 databases, which also included grey literature, there is a possibility that they might have overlooked studies related to this topic if they did not appear in their search results. Furthermore, their inclusion criteria required studies to be published in English, which could potentially introduce selection bias. Additionally, owing to the extensive diversity in study designs and outcome measurements used to assess quantitative results, only a limited subset of studies reporting findings utilising the same measure could be included in their meta-analysis.

McLaughlin and Hamilton (2019) explored the experiences of a group of former Australian military personnel with PTSD who had been matched with a service dog. Their goal was to gain insights into how the service dog affected their ability to manage PTSD symptoms and engage in significant daily activities. Their study adds to the growing body of research highlighting the potential positive benefits of partnering with a service dog for veterans with PTSD. Despite the insights collected, their results were based on a small sample.

Nieforth et al.'s (2022c) study had two key objectives. First, to outline the advantages and disadvantages of having a PTSD service dog from the perspective of veterans already partnered with these dogs. Second, to compare veterans' experiences of having a PTSD service dog against veterans who were on a waitlist for a PTSD service dog. Their study had four limitations that need to be considered. First, it was difficult to measure the therapeutic benefits of service dogs for veterans because at the time of the survey some participants had recently acquired their service dogs while others had been paired with their dogs for a significant amount of time. Second, participants were recruited exclusively from a single service dog organisation. Consequently, the results may not be easily generalisable to others enrolled in other service dog organisations with different protocols and processes. Third, selection bias may have occurred in their study as veterans with service dogs who voluntarily participated might have had more positive outcomes than those who chose not to participate. Fourth, data was collected through open-ended survey questions, which allowed veterans to express their expectations and experiences in their own words. However, this method prevented the researchers from exploring the participants' statements by asking them follow-up questions.

Richerson et al. (2023) compared the therapeutic and economic benefits of service dogs to emotional support dogs for veterans with PTSD. Their study had drawbacks, such as the absence of a control group. However, implementing a placebo-controlled design would present ethical challenges because it would involve denying a group of participants access to a potentially beneficial therapeutic option.

Rodriguez et al.'s (2020c) study had three objectives. First, to measure the significance, frequency of use, and compare PTSD symptomology of both trained and untrained behaviours exhibited by service dogs. Second, to investigate the relationship between PTSD severity, the duration since receiving the service dog, and the bond between the veteran and their dog in relation to various outcomes. Third, to compare the expectations of veterans on the waitlist for service dogs with the experiences of veterans who already had a service dog.

Despite the contributions of Rodriguez et al.'s (2020c) study, they did acknowledge that it had seven limitations. First, the results from the study could not be generalised because the participants were recruited from a single national service dog provider. Second, there may have been participation bias, with veterans who had positive experiences with their service dogs being more inclined to participate in their study. Veterans who did not have positive outcomes and who returned their service dogs to the provider were not part of the participant pool. Third, they did not measure other medications and interventions, such as psychotherapy, that the veteran participants might have been using for their PTSD. Fourth, the groups in the study were not equal in terms of all demographic variables, with more females being in the waitlist group compared to the group of participants who were already placed with service dogs. Fifth, details about the participant's race and ethnicity were not documented and the time spent on the waitlist was not considered. Since these details were not collected the researchers were unable to explain if race, ethnicity, or time spent on the waitlist had any impact upon treatment outcomes. Sixth, the researchers relied on self-reported accounts from the participants. Relying on their recollections increased the prospect of their study analysing experiences that were influenced by recall and/or expectancy biases. However, many of the factors examined in this study, such as the perceived importance of service dog behaviours and the perceived closeness with the service dog, are inherently subjective experiences. Seventh, to maximise the sample size, veterans who had recently received their service dogs were included in the sample. It is worth noting that many service dog providers suggest that veterans typically require an initial adjustment period of up to six months to establish a bond with the service dog and to fully integrate the dog into their routines and lives. Consequently, longitudinal research is necessary to gain a more comprehensive understanding of how the use and perceived value of PTSD service dogs evolve over the initial period after placement.

For their longitudinal mixed-methods study, Sherman et al. (2023) investigated the impact of *Operation K9* assistance dogs on sixteen veterans with PTSD. Their study focused on the assistance dog's influence on the veteran's inclination towards suicidality, PTSD, depression, and anxiety over a 12-month timescale, starting from the baseline assessment conducted at the time of the service dog matching. Although their study offers unique insights it does have limitations that should be acknowledged. For example, their study did not have a control group comprising veterans with PTSD who were not receiving an assistance dog. Such control groups are needed, especially when participants are required to engage in assessments over multiple time points without receiving any benefits.

The aim of Rodriguez et al.'s (2021) study was to measure the impact of PTSD service dogs on medication utilisation within a sample of military veterans who were coping with PTSD. Their study contained two limitations. First, among the participants reporting medications it was difficult to determine if medication use either enhanced, inhibited, or had no impact on the therapeutic benefits of service dog usage. Second, the sample consisted solely of post-9/11 United States veterans recruited from a single service dog provider. Therefore, the generalisability of these results to other veteran populations and/or service dog providers is unknown.

Whitworth et al. (2019) examined the efficacy of a 14-week service dog training program intended for veterans in central Florida. However, they proclaimed that their study had four limitations. First, their study lacked follow-up measures to capture data about post-completion outcomes of the service dog program. Second, the results were based on a relatively small sample size. Third, the inclusion of participant's personal dogs alongside service dogs might have influenced the results in their study.

Fourth, in their study self-reported assessment tools were used. By using such tools there is a possibility that veterans might have either exaggerated or downplayed their symptoms or tailored their responses to what they believed the researchers wanted to learn.

Shiroff et al. (2022) conducted qualitative research aimed at contributing to the existing knowledge base that advocates for the effectiveness of service dogs as an additional treatment approach for post-veterans dealing with traumatic stress disorder and/or traumatic brain injury. Despite this objective, their study had two limitations. First, all participants in this qualitative inquiry were exclusively Caucasian, married, and residing with their spouses. It would be crucial to consider exploring the perspectives of diverse ethnic groups of veterans, as well as those living independently or in homeless shelters. Second, the average duration post-service discharge was 8.3 years, and it remains unknown if the participants received medication and/or counselling alongside the use of service dogs.

3.1.2 Family Members of Veterans

The results from three studies about the impact that service dogs for military veterans had on family members were explained in the previous chapter (McCall et al., 2020; Nieforth et al., 2022a, 2022b). Nieforth et al. (2022b) assessed the influence of PTSD service dogs for veterans on their spouses and families. Despite their efforts their study had two design flaws. First, the findings from their analysis provided insights into the experiences of spouses associated with a particular service dog provider. It is conceivable that spouses from different service dog providers might have reported contrasting experiences. Second, the three-month interval between baseline and follow-up surveys might have inhibited the identification of more pronounced changes that could have emerged with a longer follow-up period. It is plausible that the service dog may not be fully assimilated into the home within three months.

While Nieforth et al.'s (2022a) study offered valuable insights into the impact of PTSD service dogs on partners of veterans, it is crucial to interpret their study's results cautiously due to two limitations. First, they recruited participants from one service dog provider. Studies in the future should explore how various service dog organisations interact with or provide training for families of veterans paired with service dogs, as this could significantly impact the reported outcomes. Second, they predominantly focused on the participant's emotional state, which is subject to various influencing factors at any given time. Emotions typically fluctuate and are interconnected with other factors. Studies in the future should consider controlling for additional variables that could influence day-to-day emotions, such as mental health diagnoses and social interactions with others.

There are a small number of studies that have explored the impacts of psychiatric service dogs on the family members of veterans, particularly their partners. McCall et al. (2020) addressed this lack of knowledge by using a mixed-methods study to collect data from 60 veteran-partner pairs. It is important to consider the limitations of this study when assessing the results. First, it is worth noting that there may be unmeasured variables, like the extent of veterans' involvement in other PTSD treatments of unobserved individual or couple-specific differences, that could have influenced their results. Second, the results were based on a relatively small sample size, even though it was relatively large for research on the effects of psychiatric service dogs. Third, those who participated in McCall et al.'s study were sourced from a single service dog provider. Given the wide variation in training methods, program structures, and participant requirements across different programs, the generalisability of their findings is limited.

3.1.3 Elderly

Salmon and Pachana (2023) reviewed the literature about the impacts of acquiring assistance dogs on various aspects of wellbeing among older adults, including practical mental, physical, and social domains. Their review also aimed to compare different types of assistance dogs and highlight potential obstacles related to obtaining these animals. However, the reliance on studies involving participants aged 50 years or more, due to a scarcity of research exclusively focused on adults aged 65 years or older, undermined their understanding about the potential impact of age as a confounding factor.

3.1.4 People with Disabilities

An examination of the results collected from the PubMed search revealed five studies about the benefits that assistance dogs gave people with disabilities (Futeran et al., 2022; Grandgeorge et al., 2023; Gravrok et al., 2020; Rodriguez et al., 2020a, 2020b). Except for Singleton's study (2023), which did not explicitly state any limitations, the limitations of these studies will be presented in this section.

Futeran et al. (2022) published a literature review of studies about the benefits that assistance dogs gave people with disabilities. To assist in achieving this outcome they used the *International Classification of Functioning, Disability and Health* framework as a guide to catalogue these outcomes. Despite including 38 studies across 41 articles there is a possibility that certain studies might not have been included in their review due to the restricted search criteria, which focused solely on papers from peer-reviewed journals published in English within the last 20 years. Consequently, non-English language studies containing potentially valuable information were excluded.

Grandgeorge et al. (2023) hypothesised that the COVID-19 lockdown might have affected the relationship between people with disabilities and their service dogs. To investigate this they administered an online survey in France during the initial phase of the COVID-19 lockdown. The findings from their study corroborates the idea that, like other pets, service dogs helped provide emotional support for people with disabilities during the COVID-19 lockdown. Despite their study's contribution to knowledge it does have three design flaws. First, the abrupt implementation of the COVID-19 lockdown prevented the researchers from collecting data before and during the lockdown. Instead, they gathered data retrospectively through questionnaires prompting respondents to report on two specific time points—prior to and during the lockdown. Despite this approach relying on the participant's recollection of events might undermine the accuracy of the responses. Second, their study lacked direct observations of the relationships between participants and their service dogs. Consequently, objective measures of the dogs' behaviour and welfare were absent, relying solely on self-reported assessments by the handlers. Third, the study's sample derived from a specific service dog provider, which limited the generalisability of their findings.

Currently, there is a lack of studies in which the effectiveness of assistance dogs to companion dogs in facilitating the wellbeing and success of their handler/owner are directly compared. This comparison is significant, considering that companion dogs are usually more affordable to obtain and more easily accessible than assistance dogs. Gravrok et al. (2020) attempted to address this gap in our knowledge. Despite their study's contribution to knowledge there were some limitations. Their study encountered limitations linked to the recruitment process. There were limited representations of certain types of assistance dogs, restricting comparisons among dog types. Additionally, their sample showed a greater prevalence of disabilities and a stronger perceived relationship with their dog that might be typical in the general population. This could be attributed to the recruitment strategy initially targeting people with disabilities and those with stronger bonds with their dogs being more inclined to complete such surveys. In the future studies should be designed that mitigate these design flaws.

Rodriguez et al. (2020a) assessed the impact of service dogs on the psychosocial wellbeing and markers of overall health in people living with physical disabilities or chronic conditions. Despite trying to achieve this aim they stated that their study had two limitations. First, the treatment group was non-randomised, potentially causing observed results to be influenced not solely by the introduction of a service dog but also by changes occurring naturally over time. Second, their research failed to include longitudinal data detailing individual variations in the progression of change following the adoption of a service dog. This progression is presumed to fluctuate among individuals based on diverse personal and environmental factors.

Rodriguez et al. (2020b) outlined and contrasted the anticipations and encounters associated with living alongside a mobility or medical service dog within individuals coping with physical disabilities or chronic conditions. Despite enriching our understanding in this field, the researchers acknowledged two constraints in their study. First, due to the participants recalling their experiences their findings were based on a potential selection bias. Second, the voluntary nature of the study raises the possibility that people who had more positive interactions with their service dogs were more inclined to partake and communicate their experiences compared to others.

3.1.5 People with Dementia

In the previous chapter the results of two studies about the benefits that people with dementia obtained from assistance dogs were reported (Marks & McVilly, 2020, 2023). Marks and McVilly's (2020) systematic literature review explored the evidence supporting the efficacy of trained assistance dogs as an intervention and support mechanism for people with dementia. Despite providing a synthesis of 24 studies, their systematic literature review did not incorporate non-English articles or studies that were not published on SCOPUS, Web of Science, and Google Scholar. In another study, Marks and McVilly (2023) conducted interviews with family carers spanning a period of up to two years. They discovered that beyond the positive impacts observed in people with younger onset dementia, family carers also reported numerous advantages extending to the broader family and their personal wellbeing. One limitation of this research is the relatively small sample size. Their study also operated within a confined timeframe, spanning over two years.

3.1.6 People with Mental Health Disorders

Lloyd et al. (2019) was the only study identified from the PubMed search that documented the benefits that psychiatric assistance dogs gave people with mental health disorders. Despite their study's contribution to improving our understanding about this topic they only recruited participants from one site. Consequently, the findings could not be generalised to other locations in Australia. Additionally, insights from participants were collected at one point in time via a survey. Thus, since this was not a longitudinal study the long-term impacts that people with mental health disorders obtain from interacting with assistance dogs could not be examined.

3.1.7 Autistic Children

In the previous section the results from five studies about the benefits that autistic children obtain from interacting with assistance or service dogs were presented (Agnew et al., 2024; Dollion et al., 2021, 2022; Leung et al., 2022; Tseng, 2023). While their studies have provided many benefits to our understanding of this subject, each study has its own limitations which are explained in this section.

Dollion et al. (2021) concluded that autistic children who interacted with a service dog were more inclined to look at social stimuli than non-social stimuli. However, their sample size was relatively small. Therefore, these findings need validation through replication with a larger sample to enhance data reliability and validate their results. Another limitation pertains to the preselection of autistic children for service dog placement, based in part on their initial attraction to dogs. This recruitment strategy might have minimised inter-individual differences in attraction to service dogs.

The objective of Dollion et al.'s (2022) study was to explore if the presence of a service dog affected the facial expression processing abilities of autistic children. Two sets of 15 autistic children were compared in facial expression recognition computer task, during which their eye movements were tracked using an eye-tracker. The groups were only differentiated by the presence or absence of a service dog. The findings from their study imply that regular interaction with a service dog might encourage the development of distinct visual exploration methods for processing human facial expressions. However, there are three limitations that should be addressed. First, the findings reported were derived from a relatively small pool of participants. Second, the information regarding autistic children and their families was obtained from records. However, specific details about the current presence of pets within the household or recent evaluations of autistic severity were not collected. Third, information regarding therapeutic interventions that the autistic children received before or during the study that could have influenced their understanding of facial expressions was not collected. Similarly, data regarding the socioeconomic status of the families, which might impact their investment in and access to rehabilitation activities for their child, was not collected.

Leung et al. (2022) assessed the impact assistance dogs on the quality of life, independence, and participation of families of autistics. They compared families that received an autism assistance dog (AAD) to those on a waiting list for such a dog. However, there were various factors that might have influenced the study's results, potentially causing differences from existing literature. Participants were undergoing other therapies and treatments outside of this study, likely affecting the outcomes that were measured. Additionally, most participants reported additional diagnoses, which might have influenced their functioning levels. Their study was also conducted during the COVID-19 pandemic, potentially impacting routines. Finally, participants also found difficulty using certain scales related to satisfaction and performance, as these concepts were influenced by their child's acceptance of their disability and comparisons to typically developing peers or siblings.

Tseng (2023) conducted a study involving autistic children and their families both before and after the introduction of a well-trained AAD, utilising a repeated-measures design within the same subjects. Notably, their research is pioneering in its assessment of changes in a biomarker associated with chronic stress in both autistic children and their parents. However, their research had two limitations. First, Tseng decided not to include two specific control groups, one comprised of families who applied for an AAD but did not receive one and another consisting of families from the community who did not apply for an AAD. They made this decision because of the complex and varied nature of each family's characteristics. Second, they encountered challenges due to the scarcity of qualified AAD, resulting in a smaller-than-expected sample size. Thus, the results could not be generalised.

Agnew et al. (2024) investigated how caregivers reported the impact of an assistance dog on the involvement in daily activities of children with autism and their families. Despite the benefits of their study, it does contain two limitations. First, the results of their study were based on a group of participants mostly sourced from a specific assistance dog organisation in Victoria, Australia. Similarly, despite implementing various measures to ensure the reliability of the qualitative data, data collection happened at one specific instance. Thus, the results could not be generalised to other groups or at different points in time. Second, it is important to consider the possibility of recall bias among participants when they were recalling their past experiences during the interview.

3.1.8 Parents of Children with a Disability

In the previous chapter descriptions about the experiences that parents had regarding their child with a disability using a service or an assistance dog were presented. Two studies described such experiences from the perspective of parents raising autistic children (Appleby et al., 2022; Hellings et al., 2022). The other two studies described such experiences from the perspective of parents who were raising children with different disabilities (Bibbo et al., 2019; Lindsay & Thiyagarajah, 2021). In this section a description of these studies and their limitations are outlined.

Appleby et al. (2022) described parental experiences concerning their autistic child interacting with an AAD. Eight families were enlisted from an Australian AAD program engaging in semi-structured, in-depth interviews conducted throughout the year 2017. Thematic analysis was used to examine the data collected from the interviews. However, their study had three limitations. First, there was a potential bias in volunteers, possibly resulting in more individuals with positive experiences being willing to participate compared to those with neutral or negative experiences. Additionally, some potential participants might have desired to volunteer but felt unable due to the high demands of caring for an autistic child requiring extensive support. Second, participants relied on their memory, leading some families to recall events up to eight years ago, potentially causing errors in reporting places visited before and after acquiring a dog. Third, while their study offered comprehensive insights into parental experiences, it was limited by its reliance on self-reporting and subjective measures.

Hellings et al. (2022) explained the expectations, advantages, and obstacles encountered by families of autistic children after acquiring an assistance dog. The findings revealed that owning an assistance dog positively impacted the child's self-regulation, socialisation, engagement in daily routines, and facilitated increased participation in family outings and activities. However, these results should be cautiously adopted because their study had three limitations. First, the participants were observed for a period of six months. Thus, any long-term effects of the assistance dog on the family were not examined. Second, the qualitative approach allowed for a comprehensive understanding of the lived experiences of assistance dog ownership among these families raising an autistic child. However, the findings were based on self-reports by the participants, which might have led to an overestimation of the assistance dog's impact. Third, all participants were mothers of autistic children. The experiences of fathers or partners of autistic children were not examined.

Bibbo et al. (2019) examined the effect of a service dog on the functioning of family members. Despite its contributions to our understanding of this topic, their study did have two shortcomings. First, details about the psychosocial health of the family members were not collected. Moreover, the medical and demographic details about the service dog recipients were derived from their initial applications. Thus, these details might have been outdated when they started the study. Second, the sample was comprised of people actively seeking a service dog, limiting the generalisability of the results solely to families desiring to incorporate a service dog into their household. Thus, it is crucial to recognise that not all families with a member enduring a chronic condition will benefit from a service dog.

Lindsay and Thiyagarajah's (2021) systematic review underscores the numerous advantages that service dogs offer children, youth, and their families. However, their review contains three shortcomings. First, their inclusion criteria were limited to articles that were written solely in English or French, potentially resulting in overlooking studies published in other languages. Second, the studies examined in their review originated from six distinct countries, each with varying guidelines, policies, and definitions concerning service dogs and disability rights. These inconsistencies, both within and across countries, might affect the impact of service dogs on children and youth. Third, many studies lacked explicit details regarding the service dogs' training type, extent, and the duration of ownership by people. Fourth, their review was comprised of studies reflecting diverse perspectives (e.g., youth, parents, and families), various disability types, and a wide spectrum of dog types, training durations, and formats. There also existed a multitude of diverse outcome measures in the studies, with some failing to test for or report statistical significance, which complicates the comparability of findings. Hence, caution needs to be exercised when making comparisons across these studies or drawing general conclusions based on the collected results.

3.1.9 Views of Professionals About the Usage of Assistance or Service Dogs

In the previous chapter the results in three studies about the views of professionals about the usage of assistance or service dogs were presented (Chan et al., 2022; Iong et al., 2022; Merk et al., 2021). The limitations of these studies are outlined in this section.

There is a lack of understanding about the experiences of Australian occupational therapists regarding assistance dogs and their views concerning their benefits to people with disabilities. Chan et al. (2022) attempted to address this issue. Although their study yielded some interesting results, it did have two shortcomings. First, the occupational therapists themselves volunteered to complete the survey, possibly because they were more likely to possess an interest in assistance dogs. This approach might have made the sample non-representative of all occupational therapists in Australia. Second, the survey was disseminated in a highly targeted manner to minimise the inclusion of unqualified participants or multiple survey completions by single occupational therapists. Despite this approach they were unable to verify the participant's identity or discover any multiple submissions.

Iong et al. (2022) described the level of understanding and viewpoints of Australian occupational therapists concerning assistance dogs. However, the findings were based on a homogeneous sample because they received more responses from occupational therapists in Victoria, Australia. Consequently, their findings might not accurately reflect the entire occupational therapist population across all Australian states and territories. Despite efforts by the researchers to collect data from various states, they failed to make their study diverse which inhibited the generalisability of their study's findings.

Merk et al. (2021) evaluated the familiarity that health professionals had with regulations concerning the American with Disabilities Act (ADA) and their perceptions about workplace protocols and training concerning service dogs. Although their results show that respondents needed more education about ADA service dog regulations such findings should be tentatively endorsed. Given that their study is one of the initial investigations in this topic many of their survey questions were formulated based on the small amount of existing literature. Additionally, they did not assess the reliability and validity of their survey instrument.

3.2 Conclusion

The purpose of this chapter was to present the limitations of the studies that were presented in the previous chapter. It was shown that despite the reviewed studies improving our knowledge about assistance and service dogs some were based on flawed study designs. For example, it was shown that in some studies participants recalled their experiences of interacting with dogs which could have fostered recall bias. Furthermore, in some studies the results were based on a small sample of participants.

References

Agnew, Z., Callaway, L., Lalor, A., Peart, A., & Bould, E. (2024). 'Having the dog as part of our family gives us hope': Experiences of the impact of assistance dogs on the occupational engagement of children with autism and their families. *Australian Occupational Therapy Journal, 71*(1), 18–34. https://doi.org/10.1111/1440-1630.12904

Appleby, R., Wright, S., Williams, L., & Stanley, M. (2022). Australian parents' experiences of owning an autism assistance dog. *Health & Social Care in the Community, 30*(6), e4113–e4121. https://doi.org/10.1111/hsc.13805

Bibbo, J., Rodriguez, K. E., & O'Haire, M. E. (2019). Impact of service dogs on family members' psychosocial functioning. *The American Journal of Occupational Therapy: Official Publication of the American Occupational Therapy Association, 73*(3), 7303205120p1–7303205120p11. https://doi.org/10.5014/ajot.2019.031690

Chan, K. W., Young, J., Williams, L. J., & Nottle, C. (2022). Assistance dogs in occupational therapy practice: A survey of Australian occupational therapists' experiences and recommendations. *Australian Occupational Therapy Journal, 69*(2), 129–139. https://doi.org/10.1111/1440-1630.12775

Dollion, N., Grandgeorge, M., Saint-Amour, D., Hosein Poitras Loewen, A., François, N., Fontaine, N. M. G., Champagne, N., & Plusquellec, P. (2022). Emotion facial processing in children with autism spectrum disorder: A pilot study of the impact of service dogs. *Frontiers in Psychology, 13*, 869452. https://doi.org/10.3389/fpsyg.2022.869452

Dollion, N., Toutain, M., François, N., Champagne, N., Plusquellec, P., & Grandgeorge, M. (2021). Visual exploration and observation of real-life interactions between children with ASD and service dogs. *Journal of Autism and Developmental Disorders, 51*(11), 3785–3805. https://doi.org/10.1007/s10803-021-05293-1

Futeran, N., Mackenzie, L., Wilkes-Gillan, S., & Dickson, C. (2022). Understanding the participation outcomes for persons with disability when partnered with assistance dogs: A scoping review. *Australian Occupational Therapy Journal, 69*(4), 475–492. https://doi.org/10.1111/1440-1630.12801

Grandgeorge, M., Rochais, C., Auffret, F., & Dollion, N. (2023). Service dogs and persons with disabilities: When COVID-19 lockdown changes their relationship. *Animals: An Open Access Journal from MDPI, 13*(5), 914. https://doi.org/10.3390/ani13050914

Gravrok, J., Howell, T., Bendrups, D., & Bennett, P. (2020). Thriving through relationships: Assistance dogs' and companion dogs' perceived ability to contribute to thriving in individuals with and without a disability. *Disability and Rehabilitation. Assistive Technology, 15*(1), 45–53. https://doi.org/10.1080/17483107.2018.1513574

Hansen, C., Iannos, M., & Van Hooff, M. (2023). Assistance dogs help reduce mental health symptoms among Australian Defence Force veterans and emergency services personnel: A pilot study. *Psychiatry Research, 324*, 115212. https://doi.org/10.1016/j.psychres.2023.115212

Hellings, D., Joosten, A., Hatfield, M., & Netto, J. (2022). Benefits and challenges of assistance dogs for families of children on the autism spectrum: Mothers' perspectives. *Qualitative Health Research, 32*(11), 1648–1656. https://doi.org/10.1177/10497323221111247

Iong, K. K., Bould, E., Lalor, A., & Callaway, L. (2022). Australian occupational therapists' knowledge of the purpose, scope, and funding of assistance dogs. *Australian Occupational Therapy Journal, 69*(1), 64–76. https://doi.org/10.1111/1440-1630.12770

Jensen, C. L., Rodriguez, K. E., & O'Haire, M. E. (2021). Service dogs for veterans and military members with posttraumatic stress disorder: Replication with the PTSD checklist for DSM-5. *Journal of Traumatic Stress, 34*, 221–228. https://doi.org/10.1002/jts.22587

Jensen, C. L., Rodriguez, K. E., MacLean, E. L., Abdul Wahab, A. H., Sabbaghi, A., & O'Haire, M. E. (2022). Characterizing veteran and PTSD service dog teams: Exploring potential mechanisms of symptom change and canine predictors of efficacy. *PLoS ONE, 17*(7), e0269186. https://doi.org/10.1371/journal.pone.0269186

LaFollette, M. R., Rodriguez, K. E., Ogata, N., & O'Haire, M. E. (2019). Military veterans and their PTSD service dogs: Associations between training methods, PTSD severity, dog behavior, and the human-animal bond. *Frontiers in Veterinary Science, 6*, 23. https://doi.org/10.3389/fvets.2019.00023

Leighton, S. C., Nieforth, L. O., & O'Haire, M. E. (2022). Assistance dogs for military veterans with PTSD: A systematic review, meta-analysis, and meta-synthesis. *PLoS ONE, 17*(9), e0274960. https://doi.org/10.1371/journal.pone.0274960

Leung, J. Y., Mackenzie, L., & Dickson, C. (2022). Outcomes of assistance dog placement in the home for individuals with autism spectrum disorder and their families: A pilot study. *Australian Occupational Therapy Journal, 69*(1), 50–63. https://doi.org/10.1111/1440-1630.12768

Lindsay, S., & Thiyagarajah, K. (2021). The impact of service dogs on children, youth and their families: A systematic review. *Disability and Health Journal, 14*(3), 101012. https://doi.org/10.1016/j.dhjo.2020.101012
Lloyd, J., Johnston, L., & Lewis, J. (2019). Psychiatric assistance dog use for people living with mental health disorders. *Frontiers in Veterinary Science, 6*, 166. https://doi.org/10.3389/fvets.2019.00166
Marks, G., & McVilly, K. (2020). Trained assistance dogs for people with dementia: A systematic review. *Psychogeriatrics: The Official Journal of the Japanese Psychogeriatric Society, 20*(4), 510–521. https://doi.org/10.1111/psyg.12529
Marks, G., & McVilly, K. R. (2023). Assistance dogs for people with younger (early)-onset dementia: The family carer's experience. *Animals: An Open Access Journal from MDPI, 13*(5), 777. https://doi.org/10.3390/ani13050777
McCall, C. E., Rodriguez, K. E., Wadsworth, S. M. M., Meis, L. A., & O'Haire, M. E. (2020). "A part of our family"? Effects of psychiatric service dogs on quality of life and relationship functioning in military-connected couples. *Military Behavioral Health, 8*(4), 410–423. https://doi.org/10.1080/21635781.2020.1825243
McLaughlin, K., & Hamilton, A. L. (2019). Exploring the influence of service dogs on participation in daily occupations by veterans with PTSD: A pilot study. *Australian Occupational Therapy Journal, 66*(5), 648–655. https://doi.org/10.1111/1440-1630.12606
Merk, A., Nelson, E., Provost, A., Rasch, M., Forster, L., Nottingham, K., Simon, J., & Fredricks, T. (2021). A survey on health professionals' understanding of federal protections regarding service dogs in clinical settings. *Journal of Osteopathic Medicine, 121*(3), 247–253. https://doi.org/10.1515/jom-2020-0280
Nieforth, L. O., Abdul Wahab, A. H., Sabbaghi, A., MacDermid Wadsworth, S., Foti, D., & O'Haire, M. E. (2022a). Quantifying the emotional experiences of partners of veterans with PTSD service dogs using ecological momentary assessment. *Complementary Therapies in Clinical Practice, 48*, 101590. https://doi.org/10.1016/j.ctcp.2022.101590
Nieforth, L. O., Miller, E. A., MacDermid Wadsworth, S., & O'Haire, M. E. (2022b). Posttraumatic stress disorder service dogs and the wellbeing of veteran families. *European Journal of Psychotraumatology, 13*(1), 2062997. https://doi.org/10.1080/20008198.2022.2062997
Nieforth, L. O., Rodriguez, K. E., & O'Haire, M. E. (2022c). Expectations versus experiences of veterans with posttraumatic stress disorder (PTSD) service dogs: An inductive conventional content analysis. *Psychological Trauma: Theory, Research, Practice and Policy, 14*(3), 347–356. https://doi.org/10.1037/tra0001021
Richerson, J. T., Wagner, T. H., Abrams, T., Skelton, K., Biswas, K., Illarmo, S., McSherry, F., Fallon, M. T., Frakt, A., Pizer, S., Magruder, K. M., Groer, S., Dorn, P. A., Huang, G. D., & Stock, E. M. (2023). Therapeutic and economic benefits of service dogs versus emotional support dogs for veterans with PTSD. *Psychiatric Services (Washington, D.C.), 74*(8), 790–800. https://doi.org/10.1176/appi.ps.20220138
Rodriguez, K. E., Anderson, L. M., Ott, C. A., & O'Haire, M. E. (2021). The effect of a PTSD service dog on military veterans' medication regimens: A cross-sectional pilot study. *Anthrozoos, 34*(3), 393–406. https://doi.org/10.1080/08927936.2021.1898219
Rodriguez, K. E., Bibbo, J., & O'Haire, M. E. (2020a). The effects of service dogs on psychosocial health and wellbeing for individuals with physical disabilities or chronic conditions. *Disability and Rehabilitation, 42*(10), 1350–1358. https://doi.org/10.1080/09638288.2018.1524520
Rodriguez, K. E., Bibbo, J., Verdon, S., & O'Haire, M. E. (2020b). Mobility and medical service dogs: A qualitative analysis of expectations and experiences. *Disability and Rehabilitation. Assistive Technology, 15*(5), 499–509. https://doi.org/10.1080/17483107.2019.1587015
Rodriguez, K. E., LaFollette, M. R., Hediger, K., Ogata, N., & O'Haire, M. E. (2020c). Defining the PTSD service dog intervention: Perceived importance, usage, and symptom specificity of psychiatric service dogs for military veterans. *Frontiers in Psychology, 11*, 1638. https://doi.org/10.3389/fpsyg.2020.01638

Salmon, A. J., & Pachana, N. A. (2023). A systematic review of the effect of assistance dog ownership on practical support, health, and wellbeing: Implications for older adults. *Clinical Gerontologist, 46*(5), 669–694. https://doi.org/10.1080/07317115.2022.2100728

Sherman, M., Hutchinson, A. D., Bowen, H., Iannos, M., & Van Hooff, M. (2023). Effectiveness of operation K9 assistance dogs on suicidality in Australian veterans with PTSD: A 12-month mixed-methods follow-up study. *International Journal of Environmental Research and Public Health, 20*(4), 3607. https://doi.org/10.3390/ijerph20043607

Shiroff, J. J., Gray, K., Santulli, G. M., DiDonato, S., Kelly, P. J., & Fulford, J. O. (2022). A qualitative exploration of the use of service dogs in veterans with post traumatic stress disorder and traumatic brain injury. *Psychiatric Research and Clinical Practice, 5*(2), 40–50. https://doi.org/10.1176/appi.prcp.20220029

Singleton, J. K. (2023). Benefits of being teamed with a service dog for individuals living with visible and invisible disabilities. Healthcare (Basel, Switzerland), 11(22), 2987. https://doi.org/10.3390/healthcare11222987

Tseng, A. (2023). Brief report: Above and beyond safety: Psychosocial and biobehavioral impact of autism-assistance dogs on autistic children and their families. *Journal of Autism and Developmental Disorders, 53*(1), 468–483. https://doi.org/10.1007/s10803-021-05410-0

Whitworth, J. D., Scotland-Coogan, D., & Wharton, T. (2019). Service dog training programs for veterans with PTSD: Results of a pilot controlled study. *Social Work in Health Care, 58*(4), 412–430. https://doi.org/10.1080/00981389.2019.1580238

Chapter 4
Directions for Research in the Future

4.1 Small Sample Size

Within 11 studies that were reviewed in the previous chapter it was identified that their results were based on a small sample of participants (Agnew et al., 2024; Dollion et al., 2021, 2022; Grandgeorge et al., 2023; Jensen et al., 2022; Marks & McVilly, 2023; McCall et al., 2020; McLaughlin & Hamilton, 2019; Sherman et al., 2023; Tseng, 2023; Whitworth et al., 2019). Due to small sample sizes it is difficult to generalise the results to the population. To overcome this limitation two strategies can be implemented. First, more participants can be recruited into the study by getting more than one or a few dog training centres to approach potential participants. Second, other places for recruitment can be accessed. For example, potential participants can be recruited from other places where dogs and people with disabilities frequent, such as veterinary clinics or medical facilities. Alternatively, recruitment can also occur within the virtual realm at places such as online support groups for assistance or service dog owners. By implementing these recommendations, as well as others, it is anticipated that the sample sizes would increase and, consequently, the generalisability of the results to the population would be improved.

4.2 Self-Reporting by Participants

Within five studies the authors explained that participants self-reported their experiences to the researchers (Appleby et al., 2022; Jensen et al., 2022; Nieforth et al., 2022b; Rodriguez et al. 2020a; Whitworth et al., 2019). This act of self-reporting experiences can undermine the integrity and accuracy of the data produced. For example, some participants may embellish their recollections due to not accurately recalling past events and/or some participants may be influenced by what they believe

G. Bennett and E. Goodall, *The Role That Assistance Dogs Play in Supporting People with Disabilities*, SpringerBriefs in Modern Perspectives on Disability Research,
https://doi.org/10.1007/978-981-97-1492-6_4

the researchers wanted to know. This point was highlighted by Whitworth et al. (2019, p. 426), who explained:

> The study was also limited by the use of self-report assessment tools, which have the potential for participant bias, although an initial established diagnosis was required. There is the possibility that veterans in the study might have over or under-reported their symptoms and responses based on what they believed the researchers wanted them to report, in addition to previously mentioned concerns about shame or stigma related to reporting suicidal thoughts or sexual behavior difficulties.

To prevent participants distorting their experiences a study's design can include opportunities when researchers obtain insights from other sources, such as the family members of the participants and/or personnel who teach assistance or service dogs and who interact with the participants. Such insights can either support or disprove their recollections of participants and in doing so can improve the accuracy of the results (Whitworth et al., 2019). This point was emphasised by Whitworth et al. (2019, p. 426), who stated:

> Use of mixed method designs that included observation of participant's behaviors, perspectives from the veteran's spouses/partners, and other qualitative components could be employed in future studies to address some of these participant bias reporting concerns and provide additional insight into a more holistic view of behavior and symptom change, from a person-in-environment perspective.

4.3 Recruiting from a Single Provider

It was identified within seven studies that the assistance or service dogs were recruited from a single provider (Jensen et al., 2022; LaFollette et al., 2019; Lloyd et al., 2019; McCall et al., 2020; Nieforth et al., 2022a; Rodriguez et al., 2021, 2020b). Only relying on one provider meant that the provider's effectiveness in teaching service or assistance dogs could not be compared. Consequently, it is impossible to distinguish between effective and ineffective methods and programs for training assistance or service dogs.

4.4 Missing Data

It was identified in four studies that details that could have improved that context of the results were not collected (Bibbo et al., 2019; Dollion et al., 2022; Jensen et al., 2021; Rodriguez et al., 2020b). For example, Jensen et al. (2021, p. 227) explained:

> There were three key pieces of information omitted from data collection that may have limited model interpretations: recent or ongoing PTSD treatments, PTSD symptom severity before service dog placement, and participants' race and ethnicity. Because information was not collected on participants' other PTSD treatments, it was unknown whether other unmeasured treatment commonalities within the service dog group could have inflated the

> association between service dog presence and less severe symptoms. The lack of information on a participant's PTSD before service dog placement prevented us from controlling for prior symptom severity.

To overcome this shortcoming researchers should endeavour to collect all data that is relevant to the study. To ensure that this occurs researchers could ask potential participants what data they believe should be collected before the data collection of the study begins. Such co-design strategies between researcher and potential participants have been described (Malloy et al., 2023; Van de Velde et al., 2024).

Co-design is not a *'one size fits all'* activity. Rather, such activities need to be tailored to the participant population that is being approached for study. For example, Hosking et al. (2023) described a framework for conducting co-design activities that are culturally safe for Aboriginal health workers in the Northern Territory who were learning a hepatitis B training course. Before conducting a study researchers should be aware of any potential cultural sensitivities of the participants. If such sensitivities are discovered the researchers should find and use guides that outline how to conduct culturally appropriate co-design activities, such as Hosking et al.'s study. Failure to undertake these preparatory tasks could increase the risk of the study being discredited due to it not being culturally appropriate.

4.5 Limited Diversity Within the Sample

Within five studies the authors acknowledged that their sample was homogeneous (Chan et al., 2022; Hellings et al., 2022; Iong et al., 2022; Jensen et al., 2021; Shiroff et al., 2022). Jensen et al. (2021) claimed that there was an over-representation of male-identifying participants. Hellings et al. (2022) stated that they only interviewed mothers for their study. Chan et al. (2022) claimed that they only sampled occupational therapists based in Australia. Iong et al. (2022) admitted that within their sample they predominantly had occupational therapists from Victoria, Australia. Finally Shiroff et al. (2022, p. 48) stated:

> the participants in this qualitative study were 100% white, were all married and living with spouses, and the sample size was small with 10 participants. Consideration of diverse ethnic groups and veterans living alone or in homeless shelters would be important to explore.

This lack of diversity has meant that the results generated could not be generalised to the population. If the intention of the study is to generalise the findings to the population then it is imperative that the sample be as diverse and as representative of the population being investigated. Alternatively, if researchers are wanting to explore specific subsets within a population, such as a particular ethnic group, then they should strive to make the sample as homogeneous as possible.

Aside from gender identity, an appraisal of the collected literature failed to reveal any studies that claimed that the samples were homogeneous regarding the participant's ethnicity, socioeconomic status, intelligence, or sexual orientation. Some studies, such as Bibbo et al. (2019) and Dollion et al. (2022), were not able to explain this potential limitation because they did not collect details about the participant or their background. In the future, researchers should collect all details required to ensure the sample is representative of the population.

4.6 Inconsistent Exposure Time to Dogs

It was identified within the examined literature that the authors of two studies explained that inconsistent exposure time between the participants and their service or assistance dogs may have tainted the results (Nieforth et al., 2022b; Rodriguez et al., 2020b). Nieforth et al. (2022b) explained that at the time of distributing their surveys to the participants some had been with their dogs for many years while others had only recently acquired their service dogs. This inconsistency was also highlighted by Rodriguez et al. (2020b, p. 13) who explained that:

> A final limitation is that we did not exclude veterans who had recently received their service dogs from participation. This decision was made to both maximize sample size and variability in exploring the effects of time since service dog placement on outcomes. Many service dog providers suggest that most veterans require an initial adjustment period of up to 6 months to develop a bond with the service dog and integrate the dog into their routines and lives. Therefore, some variation observed in importance, frequency, and value of trained tasks may have been partially due to the inclusion of veterans who may have still been in this adjustment period.

To mitigate this limitation, in the future researchers could implement two approaches. First, longitudinal research can be conducted so that any distinctions between people who have had their assistance or service dogs for a while and those who have not can be corrected. Second, a study's eligibility criteria can include a clause in which only those who have used an assistance or service dog for a minimum amount of time (i.e., six months) would be eligible to participate in the study. However, as stated in the quotation above, such a criterion might prevent the size of the sample being increased to a suitable standard that allows the generalisability of the collected results (Rodriguez et al., 2020b).

4.7 Exploring the Holistic Benefits of Assistance or Service Dogs

Some studies examined for this book had a narrow focus on what constituted a beneficial outcome for people with disabilities. For example, Hansen et al. (2023) assessed the effectiveness of two Australian Post Traumatic Stress Disorder (PTSD) assistance dog programs for alleviating PTSD and mental health symptoms over a one-year duration. Such studies have not used a holistic approach to determine the other benefits that dogs can give people with disabilities, such as if using a dog is value for money compared to other support approaches. To help identify and examine the potential holistic benefits that assistance or service dogs give people with disabilities it would be advantageous to use Section 34 of the Australian Government's National Disability Insurance Scheme (NDIS) Act to determine if the support is *'reasonable and necessary'*. For a potential support to be funded by the Australian Government, via the NDIS, it must meet all six criteria in the NDIS Act, which are:

1. (1)(a) Will the support assist the participant to pursue their goals, objectives, and aspirations included in the participant's statement of goals and aspirations?
2. (1)(b) Will the support assist the participant to undertake activities, so as to facilitate the participant's social and economic participation?
3. (1)(c) Does the support represent value for money in that the costs of the support are reasonable, relative to both the benefits achieved and the cost of alternate support?
4. (1)(d) Will the support be, or likely to be, effective and beneficial for the participant, having regard to current good practice?
5. (1)(e) Does the funding or provision of the support take into account what is reasonable to expect families, carers, informal networks and the community to provide? (Agnew et al., 2024).

By using these six legislative requirements as a framework, studies in the future can be designed to determine if the assistance or service dog gives the participants other benefits, aside from a narrowly defined focus.

4.8 Conducting Follow-Up Examinations

Nieforth et al. (2022b) explained that their approach to obtaining data from participants via a survey prevented them from returning to the participants to ask for additional clarifying information. For Nieforth et al. (2022b) this limitation meant that they could only make conclusions based on the insights collected at one point in time. Similarly, Marks and McVilly (2023) acknowledged that although the participants were observed for two years a longer observation time might have yielded more reliable and comprehensive results. For Marks and McVilly this limitation meant that they could only make their conclusions based on observations over a small amount of time. To overcome these limitations researchers can conduct longitudinal research over a course of years.

4.9 Closing Remarks

The primary objective of this book was to summarise the findings in the literature about the benefits and drawbacks that dogs can give people with disabilities and people with disabilities and/or psychological and/or medical conditions. To achieve this objective four research questions were developed to help identify citations from a single PubMed search, which was conducted on 11 December 2023. Out of the 126 citations retrieved, 41 citations were deemed to answer one or more of the research questions.

The results in the collected literature showed that interacting with dogs can give people with disabilities several benefits. For example, veterans who interacted with a service dog reported reduced symptoms of anxiety, insomnia, nightmares, and depression. Additionally, interacting with these animals can also improve social engagement and relationships among veterans. The benefits that dogs give people with disabilities can also extend to their family members.

Despite the benefits that dogs can give people with disabilities and people with disabilities and/or medical and/or psychological conditions the results in the studies examined should be treated with caution. For example, it was revealed that several studies based their results on small sample sizes or that the results were based on the participant's recall of life events as opposed to more objective measures, like family members recalling the benefits that their family members obtained from dogs. These limitations were outlined in chapter three while chapter four also outlined these limitations and then proposed some potential solutions.

Overall the literature collected and examined in this book showed that dogs can give people with disabilities and their families many benefits but the current research still has several limitations which hamper the trustworthiness of the results. For example, basing results on small sample sizes that consequently prevent the generalisation of the results to the broader population. In the interests of improving the lives of people with disabilities and the quality of our research these and other limitations should be addressed by scholars in the future.

References

Agnew, Z., Callaway, L., Lalor, A., Peart, A., & Bould, E. (2024). 'Having the dog as part of our family gives us hope': Experiences of the impact of assistance dogs on the occupational engagement of children with autism and their families. *Australian Occupational Therapy Journal, 71*(1), 18–34. https://doi.org/10.1111/1440-1630.12904

Appleby, R., Wright, S., Williams, L., & Stanley, M. (2022). Australian parents' experiences of owning an autism assistance dog. *Health & Social Care in the Community, 30*(6), e4113–e4121. https://doi.org/10.1111/hsc.13805

Bibbo, J., Rodriguez, K. E., & O'Haire, M. E. (2019). Impact of service dogs on family members' psychosocial functioning. *The American Journal of Occupational Therapy: Official Publication of the American Occupational Therapy Association, 73*(3), 7303205120p1–7303205120p11. https://doi.org/10.5014/ajot.2019.031690

Chan, K. W., Young, J., Williams, L. J., & Nottle, C. (2022). Assistance dogs in occupational therapy practice: A survey of Australian occupational therapists' experiences and recommendations. *Australian Occupational Therapy Journal, 69*(2), 129–139. https://doi.org/10.1111/1440-1630.12775

Dollion, N., Grandgeorge, M., Saint-Amour, D., Hosein Poitras Loewen, A., François, N., Fontaine, N. M. G., Champagne, N., & Plusquellec, P. (2022). Emotion facial processing in children with autism spectrum disorder: A pilot study of the impact of service dogs. *Frontiers in Psychology, 13*, 869452. https://doi.org/10.3389/fpsyg.2022.869452

Dollion, N., Toutain, M., François, N., Champagne, N., Plusquellec, P., & Grandgeorge, M. (2021). Visual exploration and observation of real-life interactions between children with ASD and service dogs. *Journal of Autism and Developmental Disorders, 51*(11), 3785–3805. https://doi.org/10.1007/s10803-021-05293-1

Grandgeorge, M., Rochais, C., Auffret, F., & Dollion, N. (2023). Service dogs and persons with disabilities: When COVID-19 lockdown changes their relationship. *Animals: An Open Access Journal from MDPI, 13*(5), 914. https://doi.org/10.3390/ani13050914

Hansen, C., Iannos, M., & Van Hooff, M. (2023). Assistance dogs help reduce mental health symptoms among Australian Defence Force veterans and emergency services personnel: A pilot study. *Psychiatry Research, 324*, 115212. https://doi.org/10.1016/j.psychres.2023.115212

Hellings, D., Joosten, A., Hatfield, M., & Netto, J. (2022). Benefits and challenges of assistance dogs for families of children on the autism spectrum: Mothers' perspectives. *Qualitative Health Research, 32*(11), 1648–1656. https://doi.org/10.1177/10497323221111247

Hosking, K., De Santis, T., Vintour-Cesar, E., Wilson, P. M., Bunn, L., Gurruwiwi, G. G., Wurrawilya, S., Bukulatjpi, S. M., Nelson, S., Ross, C., Binks, P., Schroder, P., Davis, J. S., Taylor, S., Connors, C., Davies, J., & Hep B PAST partnership. (2023). "The most culturally safe training I've ever had": The co-design of a culturally safe managing hepatitis B training course with and for the aboriginal health workforce of the Northern Territory of Australia. *BMC Health Services Research, 23*(1), 935. https://doi.org/10.1186/s12913-023-09902-w

Iong, K. K., Bould, E., Lalor, A., & Callaway, L. (2022). Australian occupational therapists' knowledge of the purpose, scope, and funding of assistance dogs. *Australian Occupational Therapy Journal, 69*(1), 64–76. https://doi.org/10.1111/1440-1630.12770

Jensen, C. L., Rodriguez, K. E., & O'Haire, M. E. (2021). Service dogs for veterans and military members with posttraumatic stress disorder: Replication with the PTSD checklist for DSM-5. *Journal of Traumatic Stress, 34*, 221–228. https://doi.org/10.1002/jts.22587

Jensen, C. L., Rodriguez, K. E., MacLean, E. L., Abdul Wahab, A. H., Sabbaghi, A., & O'Haire, M. E. (2022). Characterizing veteran and PTSD service dog teams: Exploring potential mechanisms of symptom change and canine predictors of efficacy. *PLoS ONE, 17*(7), e0269186. https://doi.org/10.1371/journal.pone.0269186

LaFollette, M. R., Rodriguez, K. E., Ogata, N., & O'Haire, M. E. (2019). Military veterans and their PTSD service dogs: Associations between training methods, PTSD severity, dog behavior, and the human-animal bond. *Frontiers in Veterinary Science, 6*, 23. https://doi.org/10.3389/fvets.2019.00023

Lloyd, J., Johnston, L., & Lewis, J. (2019). Psychiatric assistance dog use for people living with mental health disorders. *Frontiers in Veterinary Science, 6*, 166. https://doi.org/10.3389/fvets.2019.00166

Malloy, J., Partridge, S. R., Kemper, J. A., Braakhuis, A., & Roy, R. (2023). Co-design of digital health interventions with young people: A scoping review. *Digital Health, 9*, 20552076231219117. https://doi.org/10.1177/20552076231219117

Marks, G., & McVilly, K. R. (2023). Assistance dogs for people with younger (early)-onset dementia: The family carer's experience. *Animals: An Open Access Journal from MDPI, 13*(5), 777. https://doi.org/10.3390/ani13050777

McCall, C. E., Rodriguez, K. E., Wadsworth, S. M. M., Meis, L. A., & O'Haire, M. E. (2020). "A part of our family"? Effects of psychiatric service dogs on quality of life and relationship functioning in military-connected couples. *Military Behavioral Health, 8*(4), 410–423. https://doi.org/10.1080/21635781.2020.1825243

McLaughlin, K., & Hamilton, A. L. (2019). Exploring the influence of service dogs on participation in daily occupations by veterans with PTSD: A pilot study. *Australian Occupational Therapy Journal, 66*(5), 648–655. https://doi.org/10.1111/1440-1630.12606

Nieforth, L. O., Miller, E. A., MacDermid Wadsworth, S., & O'Haire, M. E. (2022a). Posttraumatic stress disorder service dogs and the wellbeing of veteran families. *European Journal of Psychotraumatology, 13*(1), 2062997. https://doi.org/10.1080/20008198.2022.2062997

Nieforth, L. O., Rodriguez, K. E., & O'Haire, M. E. (2022b). Expectations versus experiences of veterans with posttraumatic stress disorder (PTSD) service dogs: An inductive conventional content analysis. *Psychological Trauma: Theory, Research, Practice and Policy, 14*(3), 347–356. https://doi.org/10.1037/tra0001021

Rodriguez, K. E., Anderson, L. M., Ott, C. A., & O'Haire, M. E. (2021). The effect of a PTSD service dog on military veterans' medication regimens: A cross-sectional pilot study. *Anthrozoos, 34*(3), 393–406. https://doi.org/10.1080/08927936.2021.1898219

Rodriguez, K. E., Bibbo, J., & O'Haire, M. E. (2020a). The effects of service dogs on psychosocial health and wellbeing for individuals with physical disabilities or chronic conditions. *Disability and Rehabilitation, 42*(10), 1350–1358. https://doi.org/10.1080/09638288.2018.1524520

Rodriguez, K. E., LaFollette, M. R., Hediger, K., Ogata, N., & O'Haire, M. E. (2020b). Defining the PTSD service dog intervention: Perceived importance, usage, and symptom specificity of psychiatric service dogs for military veterans. *Frontiers in Psychology, 11*, 1638. https://doi.org/10.3389/fpsyg.2020.01638

Sherman, M., Hutchinson, A. D., Bowen, H., Iannos, M., & Van Hooff, M. (2023). Effectiveness of operation K9 assistance dogs on suicidality in Australian veterans with PTSD: A 12-month mixed-methods follow-up study. *International Journal of Environmental Research and Public Health, 20*(4), 3607. https://doi.org/10.3390/ijerph20043607

Shiroff, J. J., Gray, K., Santulli, G. M., DiDonato, S., Kelly, P. J., & Fulford, J. O. (2022). A qualitative exploration of the use of service dogs in veterans with post traumatic stress disorder and traumatic brain injury. *Psychiatric Research and Clinical Practice, 5*(2), 40–50. https://doi.org/10.1176/appi.prcp.20220029

Tseng, A. (2023). Brief report: Above and beyond safety: Psychosocial and biobehavioral impact of autism-assistance dogs on autistic children and their families. *Journal of Autism and Developmental Disorders, 53*(1), 468–483. https://doi.org/10.1007/s10803-021-05410-0

Van de Velde, E., Van Hecke, A., Eeckloo, K., & Malfait, S. (2024). Implementing bedside handovers in mental health care: Insights from an experience-based co-design. *Patient Education and Counseling, 119*, 108051. https://doi.org/10.1016/j.pec.2023.108051

Whitworth, J. D., Scotland-Coogan, D., & Wharton, T. (2019). Service dog training programs for veterans with PTSD: Results of a pilot controlled study. *Social Work in Health Care, 58*(4), 412–430. https://doi.org/10.1080/00981389.2019.1580238

Appendix
Dataset

G. Bennett and E. Goodall, *The Role That Assistance Dogs Play in Supporting People with Disabilities*, SpringerBriefs in Modern Perspectives on Disability Research,
https://doi.org/10.1007/978-981-97-1492-6

PubMed ID	First author	Article title	Citation	Citation included in the study (Yes/No)
37998479	Singleton JK	Benefits of Being Teamed with a Service Dog for Individuals Living with Visible and Invisible Disabilities	*Healthcare (Basel)*. 2023 Nov 19;11(22):2987. https://doi.org/10.3390/healthcare11222987	Yes
37835697	Gibson M	Insights into Canadians' Perceptions of Service Dogs in Public Spaces	*Animals (Basel)*. 2023 Oct 3;13(19):3091. https://doi.org/10.3390/ani13193091	No
37816224	Vincent C	Roles and usages of neuro service dogs for caregivers living at home with persons with dementia: An exploratory comparative case study	*Dementia (London)*. 2023 Nov;22(8):1833–1861. https://doi.org/10.1177/14713012231204646. Epub 2023 Oct 10	Yes
37770415	Agnew Z	'Having the dog as part of our family gives us hope': Experiences of the impact of assistance dogs on the occupational engagement of children with autism and their families	*Aust Occup Ther J*. 2023 Sep 28. https://doi.org/10.1111/1440-1630.12904. Online ahead of print	Yes
37726917	Gerwisch K	A pilot study into the effects of PTSD-assistance dogs' work on their salivary cortisol levels and their handlers' Quality of life	*J Appl Anim Welf Sci*. 2023 Sep 19:1–13. https://doi.org/10.1080/10888705.2023.2259795. Online ahead of print	No
37685015	Bender Y	"An Aid with Soul"—Understanding the Determinants of Guide Dog-Owner Compatibility from Qualitative Interviews	*Animals (Basel)*. 2023 Aug 29;13(17):2751. https://doi.org/10.3390/ani13172751	No

(continued)

(continued)

PubMed ID	First author	Article title	Citation	Citation included in the study (Yes/No)
37638920	Vincent C	Neuro Service Dogs Impacts on Community-Dwelling Persons with Mild to Moderate Dementia and Their Caregiver	*Stud Health Technol Inform*. 2023 Aug 23;306:230–237. https://doi.org/10.3233/SHTI230624	No
37627471	Salmon AJ	Cultivating the Acceptance of Assistance Dogs in Aged Care through Deliberative Democracy	*Animals (Basel)*. 2023 Aug 20;13(16):2680. https://doi.org/10.3390/ani13162680	No
37583981	Nieforth LO	PTSD service dogs foster resilience among veterans and military families	*Curr Psychol*. 2023 Jun;42(16):13207–13219. https://doi.org/10.1007/s12144-021-01990-3. Epub 2021 Jul 7	No
37520226	Leighton SC	Service dogs for autistic children and family system functioning: a constant comparative analysis	*Front Psychiatry*. 2023 Jul 13;14:1210095. https://doi.org/10.3389/fpsyt.2023.1210095. eCollection 2023	No
37410417	Leighton SC	Psychiatric service dog placements are associated with better daily psychosocial functioning for military veterans with posttraumatic stress disorder	*Psychol Trauma*. 2023 Jul 6. https://doi.org/10.1037/tra0001543. Online ahead of print	No
37370493	De la Fuente-Moreno E	Salivary Cortisol in Guide Dogs	*Animals (Basel)*. 2023 Jun 14;13(12):1981. https://doi.org/10.3390/ani13121981	No
37293143	Shiroff JJ	A Qualitative Exploration of the Use of Service Dogs in Veterans with Post Traumatic Stress Disorder and Traumatic Brain Injury	*Psychiatr Res Clin Pract*. 2022 Dec 21;5(2):40–50. https://doi.org/10.1176/appi.prcp.20220029. eCollection 2023 Summer	Yes

(continued)

(continued)

PubMed ID	First author	Article title	Citation	Citation included in the study (Yes/No)
37259586	Richerson JT	Service Dogs for Veterans With PTSD	*Psychiatr Serv*. 2023 Jun 1;74(6):668–669. https://doi.org/10.1176/appi.ps.20230164	No
37259585	Campbell TM	Service Dogs for Veterans With PTSD	*Psychiatr Serv*. 2023 Jun 1;74(6):668. https://doi.org/10.1176/appi.ps.20230104	No
37187229	Woodward SH	Heart rate during sleep in PTSD patients: Moderation by contact with a service dog	*Biol Psychol*. 2023 May;180:108586. https://doi.org/10.1016/j.biopsycho.2023.108586. Epub 2023 May 13	No
37174519	Morwood S	Exploring the Experiences of Volunteer Assistance Dog Puppy Raisers from the Same Program at Two Australian University Campuses	*Animals (Basel)*. 2023 Apr 27;13(9):1482. https://doi.org/10.3390/ani13091482	No
37079934	Hansen C	Assistance dogs help reduce mental health symptoms among Australian Defence Force veterans and emergency services personnel: A pilot study	*Psychiatry Res*. 2023 Jun;324:115212. https://doi.org/10.1016/j.psychres.2023.115212. Epub 2023 Apr 14	Yes
36899771	Grandgeorge M	Service Dogs and Persons with Disabilities: When COVID-19 Lockdown Changes Their Relationship	*Animals (Basel)*. 2023 Mar 2;13(5):914. https://doi.org/10.3390/ani13050914	Yes
36899634	Marks G	Assistance Dogs for People with Younger (Early)-Onset Dementia: The Family Carer's Experience	*Animals (Basel)*. 2023 Feb 21;13(5):777. https://doi.org/10.3390/ani13050777	Yes

(continued)

(continued)

PubMed ID	First author	Article title	Citation	Citation included in the study (Yes/No)
36834314	Sherman M	Effectiveness of Operation K9 Assistance Dogs on Suicidality in Australian Veterans with PTSD: A 12-Month Mixed-Methods Follow-Up Study	*Int J Environ Res Public Health*. 2023 Feb 17;20(4):3607. https://doi.org/10.3390/ijerph20043607	Yes
36718602	Richerson JT	Therapeutic and Economic Benefits of Service Dogs Versus Emotional Support Dogs for Veterans With PTSD	*Psychiatr Serv*. 2023 Aug 1;74(8):790–800. https://doi.org/10.1176/appi.ps.20220138. Epub 2023 Jan 31	Yes
36670852	Mai DL	Application of an Adapted Behaviour Change Wheel to Assistance Dog Puppy Raising: A Proposed Raiser-Centred Support Program	*Animals (Basel)*. 2023 Jan 16;13(2):307. https://doi.org/10.3390/ani13020307	No
36669063	Foltin S	Current Perspectives on the Challenges of Implementing Assistance Dogs in Human Mental Health Care	*Vet Sci*. 2023 Jan 15;10(1):62. https://doi.org/10.3390/vetsci10010062	No
36496771	Salmon A	Issues Regarding the Welfare of Assistance Dogs	*Animals (Basel)*. 2022 Nov 23;12(23):3250. https://doi.org/10.3390/ani12233250	No
36174367	Woodward SH	Reading the mind in the eyes in PTSD: Limited Moderation by the presence of a service dog	*J Psychiatr Res*. 2022 Nov;155:320–330. https://doi.org/10.1016/j.jpsychires.2022.09.012. Epub 2022 Sep 21	No

(continued)

(continued)

PubMed ID	First author	Article title	Citation	Citation included in the study (Yes/No)
36139310	Weissenbacher A	Influence of Two Types of Guide Harnesses on Ground Reaction Forces and Step Length of Guide Dogs for the Blind	*Animals (Basel)*. 2022 Sep 16;12(18):2453. https://doi.org/10.3390/ani12182453	No
36129950	Leighton SC	Assistance dogs for military veterans with PTSD: A systematic review, meta-analysis, and meta-synthesis	*PLoS One*. 2022 Sep 21;17(9):e0274960. https://doi.org/10.1371/journal.pone.0274960. eCollection 2022	Yes
36118349	Byrne C	Quantifying canine interactions with smart toys assesses suitability for service dog work	*Front Vet Sci*. 2022 Sep 2;9:886941. https://doi.org/10.3389/fvets.2022.886941. eCollection 2022	No
35918827	Salmon AJ	A Systematic Review of the Effect of Assistance Dog Ownership on Practical Support, Health, and Wellbeing: Implications for Older Adults	*Clin Gerontol*. 2023 Jan-Dec;46(5):669–694. https://doi.org/10.1080/07317115.2022.2100728. Epub 2022 Aug 2	Yes
35917950	Schulz RN	Retrospective Examination of Service Dog Training Program Participation and Mental Healthcare Utilization	*Arch Phys Med Rehabil*. 2023 Feb;104(2):237–244. https://doi.org/10.1016/j.apmr.2022.07.009. Epub 2022 Jul 30	No
35895599	Jensen CL	Characterizing veteran and PTSD service dog teams: Exploring potential mechanisms of symptom change and canine predictors of efficacy	*PLoS One*. 2022 Jul 27;17(7):e0269186. https://doi.org/10.1371/journal.pone.0269186. eCollection 2022	Yes

(continued)

(continued)

PubMed ID	First author	Article title	Citation	Citation included in the study (Yes/No)
35873697	Moxon R	A Prospective Cohort Study Investigating the Behavioural Development of Bitches in a Guide Dog Training Programme Neutered Prepubertally or Post-Pubertally	*Front Vet Sci*. 2022 Jul 7;9:902775. https://doi.org/10.3389/fvets.2022.902775. eCollection 2022	No
35772944	Hellings D	Benefits and Challenges of Assistance Dogs for Families of Children on the Autism Spectrum: Mothers' Perspectives	*Qual Health Res*. 2022 Sep;32(11):1648–1656. https://doi.org/10.1177/10497323221111247. Epub 2022 Jun 30	Yes
35668968	Dollion N	Emotion Facial Processing in Children With Autism Spectrum Disorder: A Pilot Study of the Impact of Service Dogs	*Front Psychol*. 2022 May 20;13:869452. https://doi.org/10.3389/fpsyg.2022.869452. eCollection 2022	Yes
35636742	Sykora D	Valuing Diversity in Dietetics: Considerations for Service Dogs at School, Internships, and the Workplace	*J Acad Nutr Diet*. 2022 Sep;122(9):1595–1599. https://doi.org/10.1016/j.jand.2022.05.020. Epub 2022 May 28	No
35608598	Suran M	Pilot Program for Veterans With PTSD to Train Service Dogs	*JAMA*. 2022 May 24;327(20):1949. https://doi.org/10.1001/jama.2022.7450	No
35599765	van Houtert EAE	The Impact of Service Dogs on Military Veterans and (Ex) First Aid Responders With Post-traumatic Stress Disorder	*Front Psychiatry*. 2022 May 4;13:834291. https://doi.org/10.3389/fpsyt.2022.834291. eCollection 2022	Yes
35572392	Nieforth LO	Posttraumatic stress disorder service dogs and the wellbeing of veteran families	*Eur J Psychotraumatol*. 2022 May 9;13(1):2062997. https://doi.org/10.1080/20008198.2022.2062997. eCollection 2022	Yes

(continued)

(continued)

PubMed ID	First author	Article title	Citation	Citation included in the study (Yes/No)
35470459	Futeran N	Understanding the participation outcomes for persons with disability when partnered with assistance dogs: A scoping review	*Aust Occup Ther J*. 2022 Aug;69(4):475–492. https://doi.org/10.1111/1440-1630.12801. Epub 2022 Apr 25	Yes
35439705	Nieforth LO	Quantifying the emotional experiences of partners of veterans with PTSD service dogs using ecological momentary assessment	*Complement Ther Clin Pract*. 2022 Aug;48:101590. https://doi.org/10.1016/j.ctcp.2022.101590. Epub 2022 Apr 12	Yes
35352418	Appleby R	Australian parents' experiences of owning an autism assistance dog	*Health Soc Care Community*. 2022 Nov;30(6):e4113-e4121. https://doi.org/10.1111/hsc.13805. Epub 2022 Mar 29	Yes
35175084		"Expectations versus experiences of veterans with posttraumatic stress disorder (PTSD) service dogs: An inductive conventional content analysis": Correction to Nieforth et al. (2022)	*Psychol Trauma*. 2022 Mar;14(3):376. https://doi.org/10.1037/tra0001256	No
35120413	van Houtert EAE	Hair Cortisol in Service Dogs for Veterans with Post-traumatic Stress Disorder Compared to Companion Dogs (Canis Familiaris)	*J Appl Anim Welf Sci*. 2023 Oct-Dec;26(4):623–633. https://doi.org/10.1080/10888705.2022.2033119. Epub 2022 Feb 4	No

(continued)

(continued)

PubMed ID	First author	Article title	Citation	Citation included in the study (Yes/No)
34984639	Tseng A	Brief Report: Above and Beyond Safety: Psychosocial and Biobehavioral Impact of Autism-Assistance Dogs on Autistic Children and their Families	*J Autism Dev Disord*. 2023 Jan;53(1):468–483. https://doi.org/10.1007/s10803-021-05410-0. Epub 2022 Jan 4	Yes
34944143	McManus B	Interactions between the Public and Assistance Dog Handlers and Trainers	*Animals (Basel)*. 2021 Nov 24;11(12):3359. https://doi.org/10.3390/ani11123359	No
34825714	Chan KW	Assistance dogs in occupational therapy practice: A survey of Australian occupational therapists' experiences and recommendations	*Aust Occup Ther J*. 2022 Apr;69(2):129–139. https://doi.org/10.1111/1440-1630.12775. Epub 2021 Nov 25	Yes
34819411	Takanosu M	Genotype frequency of ATP7A and ATP7B mutation-related copper-associated hepatitis in a Japanese guide dog Labrador retriever population	*J Vet Med Sci*. 2022 Jan 7;84(1):16–19. https://doi.org/10.1292/jvms.21-0369. Epub 2021 Nov 23	No
34679787	Lloyd J	Handlers' Expectations and Perceived Compatibility regarding the Partnership with Their First Guide Dogs	*Animals (Basel)*. 2021 Sep 22;11(10):2765. https://doi.org/10.3390/ani11102765	No
34602630	Groleau M	Veterinarians are well prepared for guide dog fostering	*Can Vet J*. 2021 Oct;62(10):1043–1044	No

(continued)

(continued)

PubMed ID	First author	Article title	Citation	Citation included in the study (Yes/No)
34595574	Dollion N	Visual Exploration and Observation of Real-Life Interactions Between Children with ASD and Service Dogs	*J Autism Dev Disord*. 2021 Nov;51(11):3785–3805. https://doi.org/10.1007/s10803-021-05293-1. Epub 2021 Sep 30	Yes
34573561	Mengoli M	Neurohormonal Profiles of Assistance Dogs Compared to Pet Dogs: What Is the Impact of Different Lifestyles?	*Animals (Basel)*. 2021 Sep 3;11(9):2594. https://doi.org/10.3390/ani11092594	No
34570689	McCool KE	Evaluation of Veterinary Students' Communication Skills with a Service Dog Handler in a Simulated Client Scenario	*J Vet Med Educ*. 2021 Oct;48(5):538–548. https://doi.org/10.3138/jvme.2019-0140	No
34562917	Perkins H	Immunosensor for Assessing the Welfare of Trainee Guide Dogs	*Biosensors (Basel)*. 2021 Sep 9;11(9):327. https://doi.org/10.3390/bios11090327	No
34545587	Iong KK	Australian occupational therapists' knowledge of the purpose, scope, and funding of assistance dogs	*Aust Occup Ther J*. 2022 Feb;69(1):64–76. https://doi.org/10.1111/1440-1630.12770. Epub 2021 Sep 20	Yes
34498767	Leung JY	Outcomes of assistance dog placement in the home for individuals with autism spectrum disorder and their families: A pilot study	*Aust Occup Ther J*. 2022 Feb;69(1):50–63. https://doi.org/10.1111/1440-1630.12768. Epub 2021 Sep 9	Yes
34370794	Rodriguez KE	Correction: The effects of assistance dogs on psychosocial health and wellbeing: A systematic literature review	*PLoS One*. 2021 Aug 9;16(8):e0256071. https://doi.org/10.1371/journal.pone.0256071. eCollection 2021	No

(continued)

(continued)

PubMed ID	First author	Article title	Citation	Citation included in the study (Yes/No)
34280749	Lection J	Incidence and risk factors for canine mastitis and metritis in two guide dog populations	*Anim Reprod* Sci. 2021 Aug;231:106802. https://doi.org/10.1016/j.anireprosci.2021.106802. Epub 2021 Jul 7	No
34264702	Woodward SH	Tracking positive and negative affect in PTSD inpatients during a service dog intervention	*J Consult Clin Psychol*. 2021 Jun;89(6):551–562. https://doi.org/10.1037/ccp0000572	Yes
34140755	Rodriguez KE	The Effect of a PTSD Service Dog on Military Veterans' Medication Regimens: A Cross-Sectional Pilot Study	*Anthrozoos*. 2021;34(3):393–406. https://doi.org/10.1080/08927936.2021.1898219. Epub 2021 Apr 23	Yes
34137322	Gibson PE	Public Perceptions of Australian Assistance Dogs: Happier and Better Used Than Companion Dogs	*J Appl Anim Welf Sci*. 2022 Jan-Mar;25(1):18–30. https://doi.org/10.1080/10888705.2021.1931869. Epub 2021 Jun 17	No
34077328	Nieforth LO	Benefits and challenges of mobility and medical alert service dogs for caregivers of service dog recipients	*Disabil Rehabil Assist Technol*. 2023 Aug;18(6):743–751. https://doi.org/10.1080/17483107.2021.1916630. Epub 2021 Jun 2	No
33969026	Lloyd J	The End of the Partnership With a Guide Dog: Emotional Responses, Effects on Quality of Life and Relationships With Subsequent Dogs	*Front Vet Sci*. 2021 Apr 22;8:543463. https://doi.org/10.3389/fvets.2021.543463. eCollection 2021	No
33940092	Edner A	Low risk of transmission of pathogenic bacteria between children and the assistance dog during animal-assisted therapy if strict rules are followed	*J Hosp Infect*. 2021 Sep;115:5–9. https://doi.org/10.1016/j.jhin.2021.04.025. Epub 2021 Apr 30	No

(continued)

(continued)

PubMed ID	First author	Article title	Citation	Citation included in the study (Yes/No)
33919416	Mai D	Facilitators and Barriers to Assistance Dog Puppy Raisers' Engagement in Recommended Raising Practices	*Animals (Basel)*. 2021 Apr 21;11(5):1195. https://doi.org/10.3390/ani11051195	No
33909183	Lindsay S	A Scoping Review of the Benefits and Challenges of Using Service Dogs for Finding and Maintaining Employment	*J Occup Rehabil*. 2022 Mar;32(1):27–43. https://doi.org/10.1007/s10926-021-09980-9. Epub 2021 Apr 28	No
33804470	van Houtert EAE	Do Service Dogs for Veterans with PTSD Mount a Cortisol Response in Response to Training?	*Animals (Basel)*. 2021 Mar 1;11(3):650. https://doi.org/10.3390/ani11030650	No
33663994	Ramp J	Barriers to inclusion: Service dog handlers in science laboratories	*Disabil Health J*. 2021 Jul;14(3):101070. https://doi.org/10.1016/j.dhjo.2021.101070. Epub 2021 Feb 6	No
33635961	Merk A	A survey on health professionals' understanding of federal protections regarding service dogs in clinical settings	*J Osteopath Med*. 2021 Mar 1;121(3):247–253. https://doi.org/10.1515/jom-2020-0280	Yes
33630635	Nieforth LO	Expectations versus experiences of veterans with posttraumatic stress disorder (PTSD) service dogs: An inductive conventional content analysis	*Psychol Trauma*. 2022 Mar;14(3):347–356. https://doi.org/10.1037/tra0001021. Epub 2021 Feb 25	Yes
33562832	Menuge F	Early Evaluation of Fearfulness in Future Guide Dogs for Blind People	*Animals (Basel)*. 2021 Feb 5;11(2):412. https://doi.org/10.3390/ani11020412	No

(continued)

(continued)

PubMed ID	First author	Article title	Citation	Citation included in the study (Yes/No)
33496345	Gonzales KL	Folic acid supplementation does not decrease stillbirths and congenital malformations in a guide dog colony	*J Small Anim Pract*. 2021 Apr;62(4):286–292. https://doi.org/10.1111/jsap.13292. Epub 2021 Jan 26	No
33478180	Gravrok J	Erratum: Gravrok, J., et al. Beyond the Benefits of Assistance Dogs: Exploring Challenges Experienced by First-Time Handlers. Animals 2019, 9, 203	*Animals (Basel)*. 2021 Jan 19;11(1):237. https://doi.org/10.3390/ani11010237	No
33435167	Vos SJ	A Pilot Study on the Contamination of Assistance Dogs' Paws and Their Users' Shoe Soles in Relation to Admittance to Hospitals and (In)Visible Disability	*Int J Environ Res Public Health*. 2021 Jan 10;18(2):513. https://doi.org/10.3390/ijerph18020513	No
33322634	Hunt RL	Concurrent and Predictive Criterion Validity of a Puppy Behaviour Questionnaire for Predicting Training Outcome in Juvenile Guide Dogs	*Animals (Basel)*. 2020 Dec 11;10(12):2382. https://doi.org/10.3390/ani10122382	No
33299119	O'Bryan M	Family reflections: benefits for children with service dogs	*Pediatr Res*. 2021 Mar;89(4):1032–1033. https://doi.org/10.1038/s41390-020-01289-2. Epub 2020 Dec 9	No
33264370	Rodriguez KE	The effects of assistance dogs on psychosocial health and wellbeing: A systematic literature review	*PLoS One*. 2020 Dec 2;15(12):e0243302. https://doi.org/10.1371/journal.pone.0243302. eCollection 2020	No

(continued)

(continued)

PubMed ID	First author	Article title	Citation	Citation included in the study (Yes/No)
33154549	Ramp J	Service dog handlers in STEM: diversity and inclusion efforts need work to remove barriers	*Nat Rev Endocrinol*. 2021 Jan;17(1):1–2. https://doi.org/10.1038/s41574-020-00442-5	No
33090609	Jensen CL	Service Dogs for Veterans and Military Members With Posttraumatic Stress Disorder: Replication With the PTSD Checklist for DSM-5	*J Trauma Stress*. 2020 Oct 8:10.1002/jts.22587. https://doi.org/10.1002/jts.22587. Online ahead of print	Yes
33069669	Lindsay S	The impact of service dogs on children, youth and their families: A systematic review	*Disabil Health J*. 2021 Jul;14(3):101012. https://doi.org/10.1016/j.dhjo.2020.101012. Epub 2020 Oct 11	Yes
33019025	Williams E	A Smart Collar for Assessment of Activity Levels and Environmental Conditions for Guide Dogs	*Annu Int Conf IEEE Eng Med Biol Soc*. 2020 Jul;2020:4628–4631. https://doi.org/10.1109/EMBC44109.2020.9175814	No
32849004	Rodriguez KE	Defining the PTSD Service Dog Intervention: Perceived Importance, Usage, and Symptom Specificity of Psychiatric Service Dogs for Military Veterans	*Front Psychol*. 2020 Jul 21;11:1638. https://doi.org/10.3389/fpsyg.2020.01638. eCollection 2020	Yes
32758092	McCool KE	Evaluation of Veterinary Students' Communication Skills with a Service Dog Handler in a Simulated Client Scenario	*J Vet Med Educ*. 2020 Aug 6:e20190140. https://doi.org/10.3138/jvme-2019-0140. Online ahead of print	No

(continued)

(continued)

PubMed ID	First author	Article title	Citation	Citation included in the study (Yes/No)
32734029	Ando I	Evaluation of stress status using the stress map for guide dog candidates in the training stage using variations in the serum cortisol with nerve growth factor and magnesium ions	*Vet Anim Sci*. 2020 Jun 26;10:100129. https://doi.org/10.1016/j.vas.2020.100129. eCollection 2020 Dec	No
32719570	Bray EE	Cognitive characteristics of 8- to 10-week-old assistance dog puppies	*Anim Behav*. 2020 Aug;166:193–206. https://doi.org/10.1016/j.anbehav.2020.05.019. Epub 2020 Jul 14	No
32325673	Ogi A	Effects of Stroking on Salivary Oxytocin and Cortisol in Guide Dogs: Preliminary Results	*Animals (Basel)*. 2020 Apr 18;10(4):708. https://doi.org/10.3390/ani10040708	No
32154281	Patterson-Kane E	Editorial: Assistance Dogs for People With Disabilities	*Front Vet Sci*. 2020 Feb 21;7:87. https://doi.org/10.3389/fvets.2020.00087. eCollection 2020	No
32078779	Gravrok J	The influence of contextual factors on an individual's ability to work with an assistance dog	*Disabil Rehabil*. 2021 Oct;43(21):3041–3051. https://doi.org/10.1080/09638288.2020.1728399. Epub 2020 Feb 20	No
32065698	Marks G	Trained assistance dogs for people with dementia: a systematic review	*Psychogeriatrics*. 2020 Jul;20(4):510–521. https://doi.org/10.1111/psyg.12529. Epub 2020 Feb 17	Yes
32033129	DeYoung SE	Disaster Preparedness among Service Dog Puppy- Raisers (Human Subject Sample)	*Animals (Basel)*. 2020 Feb 4;10(2):246. https://doi.org/10.3390/ani10020246	No
31941065	Mai D	Raising an Assistance Dog Puppy-Stakeholder Perspectives on What Helps and What Hinders	*Animals (Basel)*. 2020 Jan 13;10(1):128. https://doi.org/10.3390/ani10010128	No

(continued)

(continued)

PubMed ID	First author	Article title	Citation	Citation included in the study (Yes/No)
31923779	Martin-Lemoyne V	Effects of a trained mobility assistance dog on upper extremity muscular effort during wheelchair propulsion on tiled and carpeted floors in individuals with a spinal cord injury	*Clin Biomech (Bristol, Avon).* 2020 Mar;73:28–34. https://doi.org/10.1016/j.clinbiomech.2019.12.022. Epub 2019 Dec 29	No
35316935	McCall CE	"A Part of Our Family"? Effects of Psychiatric Service Dogs on Quality of Life and Relationship Functioning in Military-Connected Couples	*Mil Behav Health.* 2020;8(4):410–423. https://doi.org/10.1080/21635781.2020.1825243. Epub 2020 Oct 14	Yes
31649944	Walther S	Geographic Availability of Assistance Dogs: Dogs Placed in 2013–2014 by ADI- or IGDF-Accredited or Candidate Facilities in the United States and Canada, and Non-accredited U.S. Facilities	*Front Vet Sci.* 2019 Oct 9;6:349. https://doi.org/10.3389/fvets.2019.00349. eCollection 2019	No
31649939	Zlotnick M	Incidence of Health and Behavior Problems in Service Dog Candidates Neutered at Various Ages	*Front Vet Sci.* 2019 Oct 8;6:334. https://doi.org/10.3389/fvets.2019.00334. eCollection 2019	No
31608293	Villalobos AE	Supportive Care for People With Disabilities as Working Partnerships With Their Assistance Dogs Are Ending: A Perspective From Veterinary Oncology	*Front Vet Sci.* 2019 Sep 25;6:309. https://doi.org/10.3389/fvets.2019.00309. eCollection 2019	No

(continued)

(continued)

PubMed ID	First author	Article title	Citation	Citation included in the study (Yes/No)
31513601	Lundqvist M	Certified service dogs - A cost-effectiveness analysis appraisal	*PLoS One*. 2019 Sep 12;14(9):e0219911. https://doi.org/10.1371/journal.pone.0219911. eCollection 2019	No
31512257	McLaughlin K	Exploring the influence of service dogs on participation in daily occupations by veterans with PTSD: A pilot study	*Aust Occup Ther J*. 2019 Oct;66(5):648–655. https://doi.org/10.1111/1440-1630.12606. Epub 2019 Sep 11	Yes
31469524	Martellucci S	Assistance Dogs for Persons with Hearing Impairment: A Review	*Int Tinnitus J*. 2019 Jan 1;23(1):26–30. https://doi.org/10.5935/0946-5448.20190005	No
31443579	Chiofalo B	Thyroid and Lipid Status in Guide Dogs During Training: Effects of Dietary Protein and Fat Content	*Animals (Basel)*. 2019 Aug 23;9(9):597. https://doi.org/10.3390/ani9090597	No
31310614	Gaunet F	Guide dogs' navigation after a single journey: A descriptive study of path reproduction, homing, shortcut and detour	*PLoS One*. 2019 Jul 16;14(7):e0219816. https://doi.org/10.1371/journal.pone.0219816. eCollection 2019	No
31294038	Takayanagi T	The Use of Service Dogs for People With Physical Disabilities in Japan in Accordance With the Act on Assistance Dogs for Physically Disabled Persons	*Front Vet Sci*. 2019 Jun 21;6:198. https://doi.org/10.3389/fvets.2019.00198. eCollection 2019	No
31284677	Glenk LM	Perceptions on Health Benefits of Guide Dog Ownership in an Austrian Population of Blind People with and without a Guide Dog	*Animals (Basel)*. 2019 Jul 7;9(7):428. https://doi.org/10.3390/ani9070428	No

(continued)

(continued)

PubMed ID	First author	Article title	Citation	Citation included in the study (Yes/No)
31245394	Yamamoto M	Professionally- and Self-Trained Service Dogs: Benefits and Challenges for Partners With Disabilities	*Front Vet Sci*. 2019 Jun 11;6:179. https://doi.org/10.3389/fvets.2019.00179. eCollection 2019	No
31245389	Lloyd J	Psychiatric Assistance Dog Use for People Living With Mental Health Disorders	*Front Vet Sci*. 2019 Jun 6;6:166. https://doi.org/10.3389/fvets.2019.00166. eCollection 2019	Yes
31194832	Bogaerts E	Rejections in an non-purpose bred assistance dog population: Reasons, consequences and methods for screening	*PLoS One*. 2019 Jun 13;14(6):e0218339. https://doi.org/10.1371/journal.pone.0218339. eCollection 2019	No
31181852	Tandon D	Homozygosity for Mobile Element Insertions Associated with WBSCR17 Could Predict Success in Assistance Dog Training Programs	*Genes (Basel)*. 2019 Jun 9;10(6):439. https://doi.org/10.3390/genes10060439	No
31120842	Bibbo J	Impact of Service Dogs on Family Members' Psychosocial Functioning	*Am J Occup Ther*. 2019 May/Jun;73(3):7303205120p1-7303205120p11. https://doi.org/10.5014/ajot.2019.031690	Yes
31094574	Gravrok J	The experience of acquiring an assistance dog: examination of the transition process for first-time handlers	*Disabil Rehabil*. 2021 Jan;43(1):49–59. https://doi.org/10.1080/09638288.2019.1615561. Epub 2019 May 16	No

(continued)

(continued)

PubMed ID	First author	Article title	Citation	Citation included in the study (Yes/No)
31035674	Gravrok J	Beyond the Benefits of Assistance Dogs: Exploring Challenges Experienced by First-Time Handlers	*Animals (Basel)*. 2019 Apr 29;9(5):203. https://doi.org/10.3390/ani9050203	No
31012752	Lamontagne ME	Facilitators and barriers to the use of service dogs: an exploratory study using the Theoretical Domains Framework	*Disabil Rehabil Assist Technol*. 2020 Jul;15(5):537–544. https://doi.org/10.1080/17483107.2019.1594406. Epub 2019 Apr 23	No
30907171	Rodriguez KE	Mobility and medical service dogs: a qualitative analysis of expectations and experiences	*Disabil Rehabil Assist Technol*. 2020 Jul;15(5):499–509. https://doi.org/10.1080/17483107.2019.1587015. Epub 2019 Mar 25	Yes
30875483	Whitworth JD	Service dog training programs for veterans with PTSD: results of a pilot controlled study	*Soc Work Health Care*. 2019 Apr;58(4):412–430. https://doi.org/10.1080/00981389.2019.1580238	Yes
30873418	Bray EE	Predictive Models of Assistance Dog Training Outcomes Using the Canine Behavioral Assessment and Research Questionnaire and a Standardized Temperament Evaluation	*Front Vet Sci*. 2019 Feb 27;6:49. https://doi.org/10.3389/fvets.2019.00049. eCollection 2019	No
30859106	Grigg EK	Enhancing Success of Veterinary Visits for Clients With Disabilities and an Assistance Dog or Companion Animal: A Review	*Front Vet Sci*. 2019 Feb 25;6:44. https://doi.org/10.3389/fvets.2019.00044. eCollection 2019	No

(continued)

(continued)

PubMed ID	First author	Article title	Citation	Citation included in the study (Yes/No)
30846141	Nielson E	Who Let the Dogs Out? A Legal Primer on Service Dogs in the Emergency Department	*J Emerg Nurs*. 2019 Mar;45(2):208–210. https://doi.org/10.1016/j.jen.2018.12.015	No
30819924	Pemberton N	Cocreating guide dog partnerships: dog training and interdependence in 1930s America	*Med Humanit*. 2019 Mar;45(1):92–101. https://doi.org/10.1136/medhum-2018-011626	No
30819923	Wlodarczyk J	When pigs fly: emotional support animals, service dogs and the politics of legitimacy across species boundaries	*Med Humanit*. 2019 Mar;45(1):82–91. https://doi.org/10.1136/medhum-2018-011625	No
30805353	LaFollette MR	Military Veterans and Their PTSD Service Dogs: Associations Between Training Methods, PTSD Severity, Dog Behavior, and the Human-Animal Bond	*Front Vet Sci*. 2019 Feb 11;6:23. https://doi.org/10.3389/fvets.2019.00023. eCollection 2019	Yes
30794614	Leighton EA	Genetic improvement of hip-extended scores in 3 breeds of guide dogs using estimated breeding values: Notable progress but more improvement is needed	*PLoS One*. 2019 Feb 22;14(2):e0212544. 10.1371/journal.pone.0212544. eCollection 2019	No
30689466	Gravrok J	Thriving through relationships: assistance dogs' and companion dogs' perceived ability to contribute to thriving in individuals with and without a disability	*Disabil Rehabil Assist Technol*. 2020 Jan;15(1):45–53. https://doi.org/10.1080/17483107.2018.1513574. Epub 2019 Jan 28	Yes

(continued)

(continued)

PubMed ID	First author	Article title	Citation	Citation included in the study (Yes/No)
30634884	Rodriguez KE	The effects of service dogs on psychosocial health and wellbeing for individuals with physical disabilities or chronic conditions	*Disabil Rehabil*. 2020 May;42(10):1350–1358. https://doi.org/10.1080/09638288.2018.1524520. Epub 2019 Jan 11	Yes
32789248	Ikenaga Y	Changes in the Health Condition after Using a Service Dog of a Person with Complete C5 Spinal Cord Injury: A Qualitative Single Case Study	*Prog Rehabil Med*. 2019 Jan 1;4:20190001. https://doi.org/10.2490/prm.20190001. eCollection 2019	No
30570307	Stumbo SP	Preliminary evidence is promising, but challenges remain in providing service dogs to veterans: Commentary on preliminary efficacy of service dogs as a complementary treatment for posttraumatic stress disorder in military members and veterans (O'Haire & Rodriguez, 2018)	*J Consult Clin Psychol*. 2019 Jan;87(1):118–121. https://doi.org/10.1037/ccp0000352	No
30264598	Meyer D	Profiling guide dog handlers to support guide dog matching decisions	*Disabil Rehabil*. 2020 Jan;42(1):137–146. https://doi.org/10.1080/09638288.2018.1494211. Epub 2018 Sep 28	No
29157032	Vincent C	Pain, fatigue, function and participation among long-term manual wheelchair users partnered with a mobility service dog	*Disabil Rehabil Assist Technol*. 2019 Feb;14(2):99–108. https://doi.org/10.1080/17483107.2017.1401127. Epub 2017 Nov 20	No

Notes
Search conducted on 11 December 2023

Search terms: (*“assistance dog*”* [Title]) OR (*“service dog*”* [Title]) OR (*“support dog*”* [Title]) OR (*“guide dog*”* [Title])
Date range of citations: 11 December 2018 to 11 December 2023
Language of citations

www.ingramcontent.com/pod-product-compliance
Ingram Content Group UK Ltd.
Pitfield, Milton Keynes, MK11 3LW, UK
UKHW020704041026
15590UKWH00001B/457
* 9 7 8 9 8 1 9 7 1 4 9 1 9 *